TOPICAL STERO
FOR SKIN DISOI

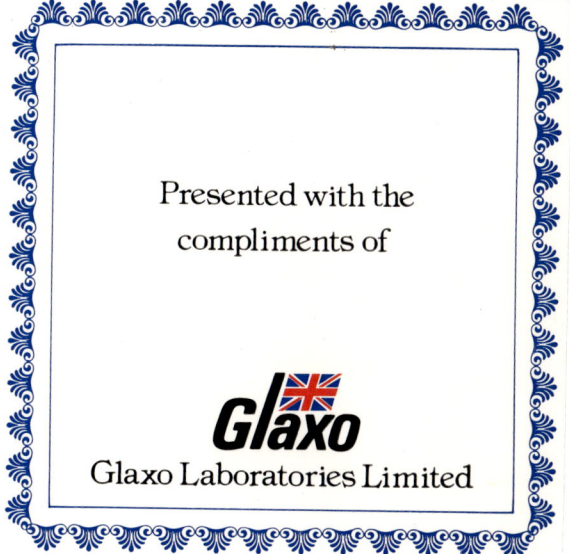

Presented with the compliments of

Glaxo Laboratories Limited

Topical Steroids for Skin Disorders

Michèle Clement, BSC MRCP
Anthony du Vivier, MD FRCP
Department of Dermatology,
King's College Hospital, London SE5 9RS

Blackwell Scientific Publications
OXFORD LONDON EDINBURGH
BOSTON PALO ALTO MELBOURNE

© 1987 by
Blackwell Scientific Publications
Editorial offices:
Osney Mead, Oxford, OX2 0EL
8 John Street, London, WC1N 2ES
23 Ainslie Place, Edinburgh, EH3 6AJ
52 Beacon Street, Boston
 Massachusetts 02108, USA
667 Lytton Avenue, Palo Alto
 California 94301, USA
107 Barry Street, Carlton
 Victoria 3053, Australia

All rights reserved. No part of this publication may be reproduced, stored in a retrieval system, or transmitted, in any form or by any means, electronic, mechanical, photocopying, recording or otherwise without the prior permission of the copyright owner

First published 1987

Set by Setrite, Hong Kong
Printed by Dah Hua Printing
Press Co. Ltd, Hong Kong

DISTRIBUTORS

USA
 Year Book Medical Publishers
 35 East Wacker Drive
 Chicago, Illinois 60601

Canada
 The C.V. Mosby Company
 5240 Finch Avenue East
 Scarborough, Ontario

Australia
 Blackwell Scientific Publications
  (Australia) Pty Ltd
 107 Barry Street
 Carlton, Victoria 3053

British Library
Cataloguing in Publication Data

Clement, Michèle
 Topical steroids for skin disorders.
 1. Skin — Diseases — Chemotherapy
 2. Steroid drugs
 I. Title   II. Vivier, Anthony du
 616.5'061   RL110

 ISBN 0-632-01344-3

Contents

Preface, vii

Acknowledgements, viii

1 Historical Perspective, 1

2 Structure—Function Relationships, 6

3 Mechanisms of Action and their Clinical Relevance, 9

4 Potency Groups of Steroids, 16

5 Correct Use as Determined by Site and Age, 21

6 Correct Use as Determined by Disease, 32

7 Side-Effects, 49

8 Practical Aspects of Prescribing, 63

Index, 70

Preface

Topical steroids have revolutionised the treatment of many common and distressing skin disorders since their introduction in the 1950s. Enthusiasm for these highly effective agents was at its peak during the 1960s and 1970s and perhaps inevitably, the more potent steroids were often used inappropriately and indiscriminately. Adverse effects became apparent and the subsequent backlash of opinion against topical steroids has created confusion among non-dermatologists concerning the correct use of these agents. In addition, the general public has been alerted to these side-effects, largely through the media, with the result that there is now considerable concern about and prejudice against all steroid-containing preparations.

This book is intended to redress the balance and to place into perspective both the therapeutic value and the problems of topical steroids. It is aimed specifically at the general practitioner for whom skin diseases comprise a significant proportion of everyday practice.

The history, pharmacology, correct use, misuse and side-effects of topical steroids are discussed. The text has been kept deliberately to a minimum with important points highlighted by tables and illustrated with clinical and histopathological pictures. The intention is to provide the busy general practitioner with an informed and practical account of the place of topical steroids in dermatology.

Michèle Clement
Anthony du Vivier

Acknowledgements

The authors wish to thank Dr Phillip McKee for his advice and for the excellent histopathological photomicrographs; Dr David Atherton for the photograph of infantile gluteal granulomata, the Photographic Department of King's College Hospital for producing many of the other clinical photographs and Mrs P. Rowden for so patiently typing the many drafts of the manuscript.

Chapter 1
Historical Perspective

The introduction of cortisone and corticotropin for the treatment of rheumatoid arthritis by Hench *et al.* in 1949 also proved to be a major landmark for dermatology (Kierland *et al.* 1952). Prior to this there had been no effective treatment for conditions such as eczema, lichen planus and discoid lupus erythematosus and the effectiveness of systemic steroid therapy in clearing these diseases naturally led to a search for steroids which would be active when applied topically.

Hydrocortisone was the first of these but its usefulness was confined to the treatment of mild eczema (Sulzberger & Witten 1952; Sulzberger, Witten & Smith 1953). A period of intensive research by the pharmaceutical industry produced more effective products. These increases in topical potency were achieved by modification of the structure of the cortisol molecule (*see* Chapter 2). The first of the more potent products were fluocinolone acetonide and triamcinolone acetonide; the latter was found to have an anti-inflammatory effect 40 times that of hydrocortisone in animal studies and to be more effective than 1% hydrocortisone in the treatment of eczema in double-blind clinical trials (Smith, Zawisza & Blank 1958; Polano 1961). These two products became regarded as the standards for comparison for the numerous topical steroids subsequently produced.

Progress in finding topical steroids of greater potency was slow, largely because of the unreliability of laboratory screening tests for topical activity. In 1962 McKenzie & Stoughton reported a new assay which was practical and reliable and this

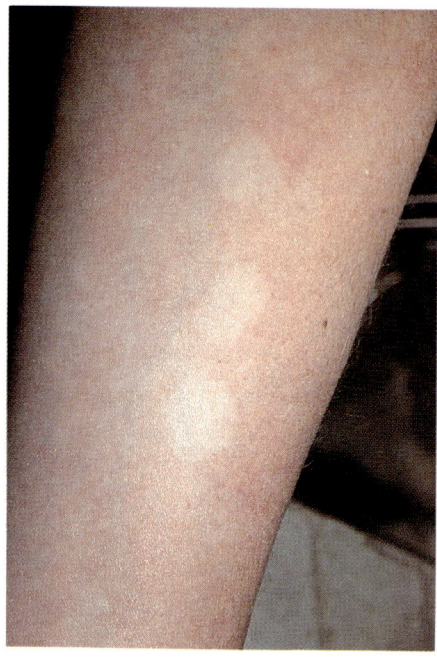

Fig. 1.1 Areas of blanching produced by the vasoconstricting action of a potent topical steroid applied to normal forearm skin.

enabled new derivatives to be assessed rapidly and effectively. The basis of this assay was the observation that corticosteroids, dissolved in alcohol and applied to normal human skin, produce areas of vasoconstriction (Fig. 1.1). Although the relevance of this vasoconstriction to the therapeutic action of topical steroids is obscure, in general it follows that the greater the degree of blanching the greater the therapeutic efficacy of the steroid.

The next important development in topical steroid therapy arose as a direct result of this vasoconstrictor assay. Several thousand vasoconstrictor tests on about 50 newly synthesised corticosteroids revealed one compound with more than three times the vasoconstricting power of fluocinolone acetonide (McKenzie & Atkinson 1964). This compound, betamethasone 17-valerate, (Betnovate), was subsequently tested in a large multicentre, double-blind trial (Williams *et al.* 1964). It was found to be more effective than five other topical steroids in the treatment of eczema and psoriasis and this discovery of a topical steroid effective in psoriasis was a major breakthrough in dermatological therapy. With reports of increases in potency of topical steroids by polythene occlusion (Sulzberger & Witten 1961), it became routine practice during the 1960s for patients with psoriasis to be treated by daily application of betamethasone 17-valerate followed by total body polythene occlusion with plastic suits. This produced a new and effective treatment for psoriasis although it soon became apparent that the improvement was temporary, with a rapid and often severe relapse of the psoriasis once treatment was stopped.

During the 1960s and early 1970s many more topical steroids of similar potency to betamethasone 17-valerate were marketed, but in 1974 the effects of a new, extremely potent steroid, clobetasol propionate (Dermovate) were reported (Sparkes & Wilson 1974). This drug proved to be considerably more effective than betamethasone 17-valerate in psoriasis and obviated the need for tiresome occlusive techniques.

The undoubted efficacy of these topical steroids, particularly in such common and troublesome diseases as eczema and psoriasis, meant that they were used indiscriminately during this time. Many doctors were prescribing them for the wrong conditions or were prescribing preparations too potent for the site or condition being treated and patients were applying the steroids in excessive quantities. Gradually, reports of local side-effects began to emerge and, with the widespread use of clobetasol propionate, potentially serious systemic effects such as Cushing's syndrome were being recorded (*see* Chapter 7).

These adverse effects of the potent topical steroids were widely publicised in the medical literature and in the lay press and a reversal in the attitude to their use took place. This continues to the present day among both the general public and many general practitioners with the result that the therapeutic potential of these invaluable agents is often not fully realised in clinical practice. Now, with the benefit of many years of experience with these potent products, it is possible to view the adverse effects in proportion and to lay down practical guidelines for safe and effective topical steroid therapy.

REFERENCES

Hench P.S., Kendall E.C., Slocumb C.H. & Polley H.F. (1949). The effect of a hormone of the adrenal cortex (17-hydroxy-11-dehydrocorticosterone) and of pituitary adrenocorticotropic hormone on rheumatoid arthritis: preliminary report. *Proc Staff Meet, Mayo Clin* **24**: 181.

Kierland R.R., O'Leary P.A., Brunsting L.A. & Didcot J.W. (1952). Cortisone and corticotropin (ACTH) in dermatology. *JAMA* **148**: 23.

McKenzie A.W. & Stoughton R.B. (1962). Method for comparing percutaneous absorption of steroids. *Arch Dermatol* **86**: 608.

McKenzie A.W. & Atkinson R.M. (1964). Topical activities of betamethasone esters in man. *Arch Dermatol* **89**: 741.

Polano M.K. (1961). Triamcinolone acetonide cream in a double-blind test. *Arch Dermatol* **83**: 214.

Smith J.G., Zawisza R.J. & Blank H. (1958). Triamcinolone acetonide: a highly effective new topical steroid. *Arch Dermatol* **78**: 643.

Sparkes C.G. & Wilson L. (1974). The clinical evaluation of a new topical steroid, clobetasol propionate. *Br J Dermatol* **90**: 197.

Sulzberger M.B. & Witten V.H. (1952). The effect of topically applied Compound F in selected dermatoses. *J Invest Dermatol* **19**: 101.

Sulzberger M.B. & Witten V.H. (1961). Thin pliable plastic films in topical dermatologic therapy. *Arch Dermatol* **84**: 1027.

Sulzberger M.B., Witten V.H. & Smith C. (1953). Hydrocortisone (Compound F) acetate ointment in dermatological therapy. *JAMA*. **151**: 468.

Williams D.I., Wilkinson D.S., Overton J., Milne J.A., McKenna W.B., Lyell A. & Church R. (1964). Betamethasone 17-valerate: a new topical corticosteroid. *Lancet* **i**: 1177.

MAJOR HISTORICAL LANDMARKS

1949   Cortisone and corticotropin for systemic use

1952   Topical hydrocortisone effective in eczema

1958   Fluocinolone acetonide and triamcinolone acetonide (fluorinated corticosteroids) introduced

1964   Betamethasone 17-valerate: effective in psoriasis

1974   Clobetasol propionate: a very potent topical steroid

Chapter 2
Structure−Function Relationships

An effective topical steroid compound must not only have inherent glucocorticosteroid activity but must also be able to pass through the stratum corneum. Early research with corticosteroids concentrated on increasing the inherent activity of cortisol, producing compounds initially for systemic use but which were later modified for topical use.

Modifications of the basic steroid skeleton and cortisone, which is inactive topically, are shown in Fig. 2.1. Reduction of the oxo group at the 11 position results in hydrocortisone which has topical activity. Insertion of a double bond at the 1, 2 posi-

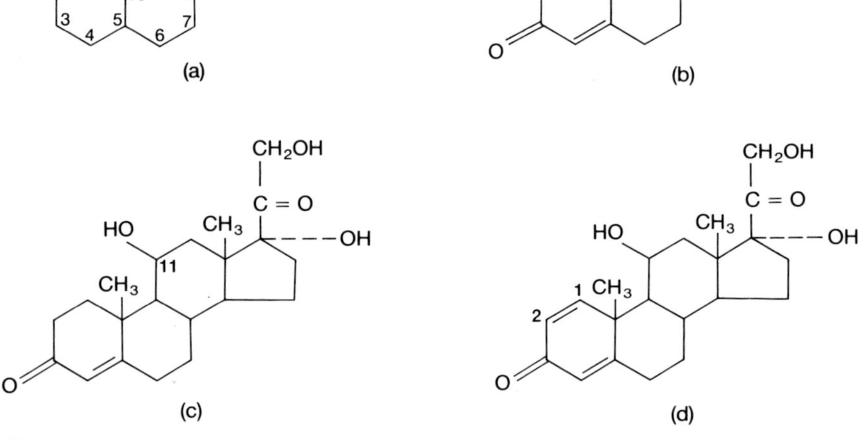

Fig. 2.1 Modification of the basic steroid skeleton (a); resulting in (b) cortisone; (c) hydrocortisone; and (d) prednisolone.

tion produces prednisolone which has greater activity than hydrocortisone. The inherent activity of hydrocortisone and prednisolone can be further enhanced by fluorination at the 6 and/or 9 positions. The 9 α-fluoro substitution, however, results in unwanted mineralocorticoid effects, even from topical application but these can be eliminated by α-hydroxyl, α-methyl or β-methyl substitutions at the 16 position. Thus, for example, modification of prednisolone by 16 α-hydroxylation and 9 α-fluorination results in triamcinolone and by 16 β-methylation and 9 α-fluorination produces betamethasone.

Other modifications to the steroid structure which are particularly important for topical activity (Fig. 2.2) are esterification at the 16, 17 or 21 positions, creating steroid esters, or the addition of a 16 α-hydroxy substituent, thereby producing an acetonide. These modifications increase the lipophilic nature of

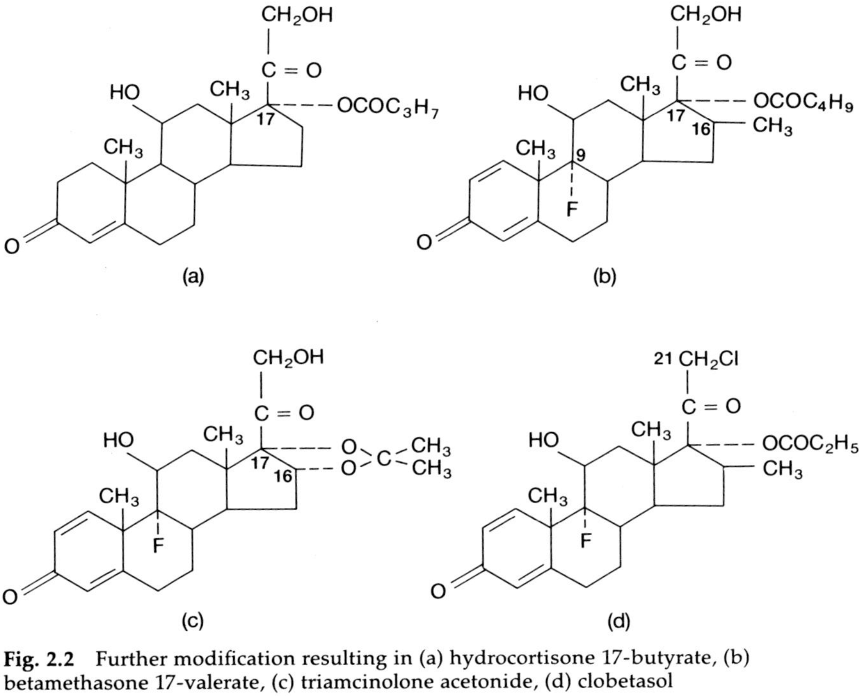

Fig. 2.2 Further modification resulting in (a) hydrocortisone 17-butyrate, (b) betamethasone 17-valerate, (c) triamcinolone acetonide, (d) clobetasol 17-propionate.

the steroids and hence their solubility in the stratum corneum by masking the hydrophilic hydroxyl groups. Thus esterification of hydrocortisone with butyric acid at the 17 position results in hydrocortisone butyrate which is considerably more effective than hydrocortisone, falling in the same potency group as triamcinolone and fluocinolone. Betamethasone alcohol is highly potent systemically but has little topical activity. Its esters, however, such as betamethasone 17-valerate and betamethasone 17-21-dipropionate, being relatively more lipophilic, are potent topical steroids. Similarly the acetonides such as triamcinolone acetonide and fluocinolone acetonide are far more active topically than the basic steroid compound.

The most potent topical steroid available, clobetasol propionate, is a derivative of betamethasone made by 21-chlorination of 21-desoxybetamethasone 17-propionate.

A further important determinant of topical steroid activity is the stability and solubility of the steroid in its vehicle and the solubility of the vehicle in the stratum corneum. Most of the steroid preparations currently available contain propylene glycol and/or isopropyl myristate as vehicles which combine efficacy with acceptability.

MODIFICATIONS OF THE BASIC STEROID SKELETON WHICH PRODUCES EFFECTIVE TOPICAL STEROIDS

- Reduction of oxo group at 11
- Insertion of double bond at 1, 2
- Fluorination at 6 and/or 9
- Hydroxylation/methylation at 16
- Esterification at 16, 17 or 21
- Addition of 16 α-hydroxy substituent

Chapter 3
Mechanisms of Action and their Clinical Relevance

Topical steroids have four main effects on the skin: anti-inflammatory, immunosuppressive, anti-mitotic and vasoconstrictive. The precise cellular and subcellular events which produce these actions are still the subject of research but there are now a number of well established facts relating to the mechanism of action of glucocorticoids.

THE ACTION OF STEROIDS AT A MOLECULAR LEVEL

Specific cytoplasmic receptors bind the glucocorticoid after it has penetrated the cell membrane. These receptors have been demonstrated in all target tissues including skin (Epstein & Bonifas 1982). The steroid-receptor complex is then translocated to the nucleus, interacts with a nuclear binding site and induces de novo mRNA transcription which produces new protein (Gorski & Gannon 1976). Hence glucocorticoids modify gene expression and act as inducers of new protein synthesis in their target organs. In some tissues they stimulate the synthesis of inhibitory proteins and hence produce a catabolic effect. The glucocorticoids also appear to have a 'permissive' effect for the actions of many other hormones by inducing enzymes which are subsequently activated by cyclic AMP.

Anti-inflammatory effects

Corticosteroids suppress the manifestations of inflammation whether the provoking agent is infectious, immunological, radiant, mechanical or chemical. They inhibit many aspects of the inflammatory response: probably their most significant actions are the reduction of neutrophil and monocyte recruitment into the affected area (Parrillo & Fauci 1979) and the suppression of the response of macrophages to macrophage migration inhibitory factor so that macrophages do not accumulate locally (Balow & Rosenthal 1973).

It has been demonstrated (Blackwell et al. 1978) that, by inhibiting phospholipase A_2, the glucocorticoids prevent the cellular biosynthesis of arachidonic acid and hence of the powerful proinflammatory mediators prostaglandins, leukotrienes and hydroxyacids. This reduction in arachidonic acid had previously been demonstrated in psoriatic skin (Hammarström et al. 1977). Furthermore it has been shown that the anti-phospholipase effect is exerted by proteins ('second messenger' polypeptides) which are synthesised by and released from target cells in the presence of the steroid (Blackwell et al. 1982). Two such proteins have now been described and named lipomodulin and macrocortin. It has not yet been established whether these are separate entities or whether macrocortin is in fact a breakdown product of lipomodulin (Fig. 3.1). This reduction in compounds known to be instrumental in chemotaxis and inflammation certainly accounts for some of the anti-inflammatory properties of the corticosteroids.

Immunosuppressive effects

Since immunological events can incite inflammatory reactions, it is obvious that there is considerable overlap between the anti-inflammatory and immunosuppressive effects of corticosteroids. In addition, however, it is well known that the cell-mediated immune reaction (delayed hypersensitivity) can be suppressed by corticosteroids. With particular relevance to the skin, it has been demon-

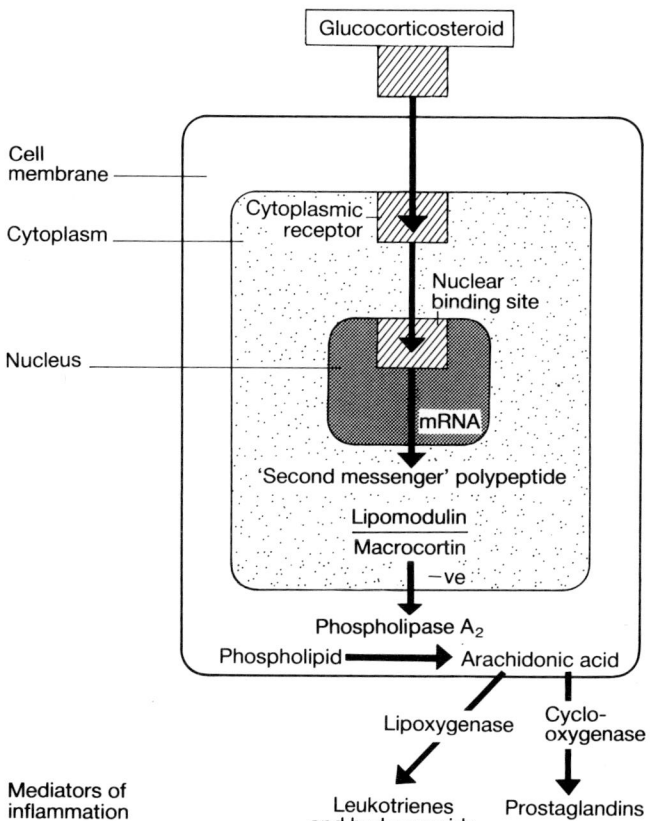

Fig. 3.1 Proposed mechanism accounting for some of the anti-inflammatory effects of glucocorticosteroids.

strated that topical steroids inhibit the development of sensitisation to topically applied dinitrochlorobenzene (Burrows & Stoughton 1976). The exact mechanism by which this is accomplished is not clear but T-lymphocytes which are the cells directly concerned in cell-mediated immunity appear to be more sensitive to the inhibitory effects of corticosteroids than the B-lymphocytes (Claman 1972).

Anti-mitotic effects

It is likely that the steroid-genome interaction discussed above is responsible for the anti-mitotic effects of the glucocorticoids. Inhibition of epidermal DNA synthesis is well documented following topical steroid application although doubt still exists as to the exact phase in the cell cycle at which the steroid acts. There is evidence of inhibition in both the G_1 and the G_2 phases but it is also possible that a general reduction in macromolecular synthesis results in a non cell-cycle-specific inhibition of mitosis.

Vasoconstrictive effects

There are probably several mechanisms underlying the vasoconstrictive actions of the glucocorticoids. The inhibition of prostaglandin formation undoubtedly plays a part since, in general, prostaglandins are vasodilators. Inhibition of the action of histamine and vasoactive kinins, potentiation of the vasoconstricting action of adrenaline by the 'permissive' effect of steroids mentioned earlier, and a direct action on vascular endothelial cells, may also be involved. The vasoconstrictive effects of steroids contribute to their anti-inflammatory properties.

CLINICAL RELEVANCE OF THE MECHANISMS OF ACTION

In practice, it is chiefly for their *anti-inflammatory and immunosuppressive* effects that topical steroids are used in dermatology. They produce a beneficial symptomatic response in inflammatory conditions such as acute sunburn and severe insect bite reactions. Conditions in which the aetiology is known to comprise a strong immunological component, such as lichen planus (Fig. 3.2), and autoimmune disorders, such as discoid lupus erythematosus, also respond well to treatment with topical steroids of the appropriate potency. In some conditions, e.g. eczema, there is an overlap between the immunological and inflammatory processes and here topical steroids are particularly useful. Despite their effects

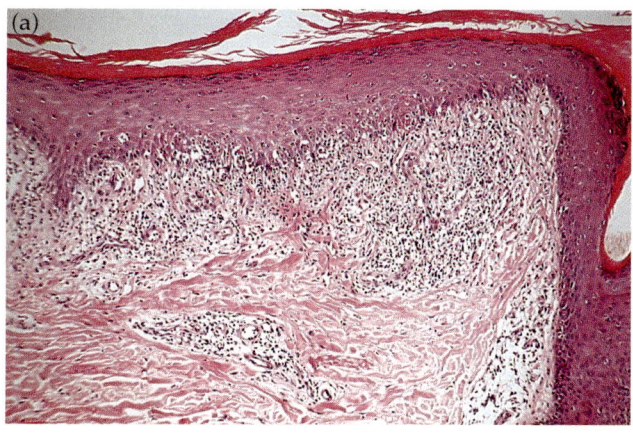

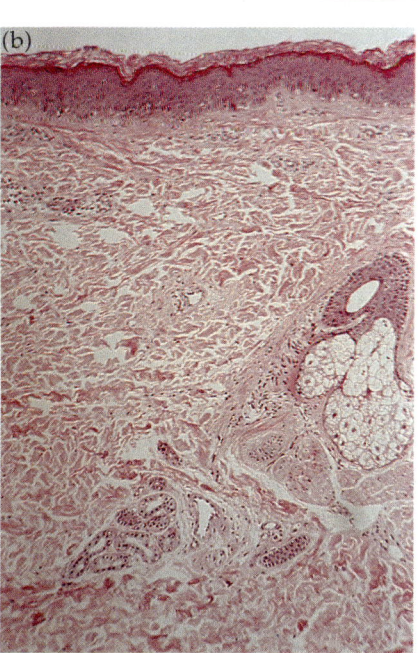

Fig. 3.2 (a) Histology of lichen planus (H & E × 30 approx.), with (b) normal forearm skin (H & E × 30 approx.) to compare. The heavy lymphohistiocytic infiltrate in the upper dermis in lichen planus is indicative of marked immunological activity.

on prostaglandins and other vasoactive mediators in the skin, topical steroids are of no value in the treatment of urticaria, angio-oedema or of pruritus with no demonstrable cutaneous cause.

The beneficial effect of topical steroids in psoriasis is probably largely the result of their *anti-mitotic effects* (Fig. 3.3) although the anti-inflammatory

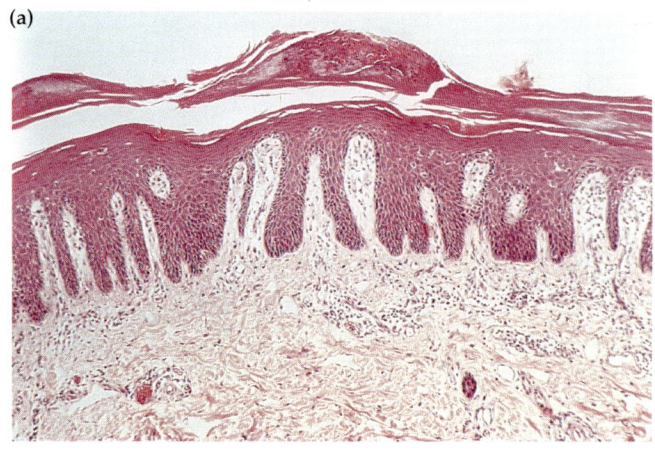

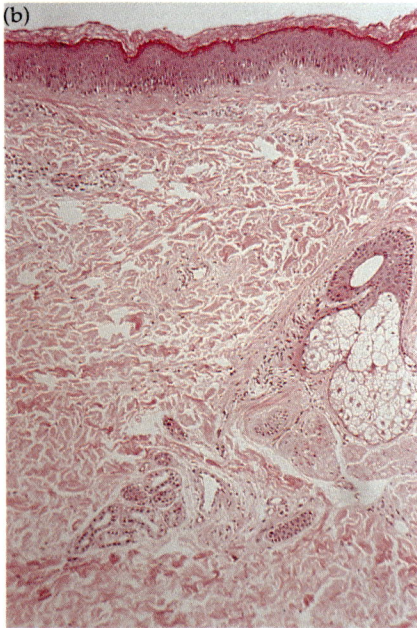

Fig. 3.3 (a) Histology of psoriasis (H & E × 30 approx.), with (b) normal forearm skin to compare. The hyperkeratosis and elongation of the rete ridges reflect the increased mitotic rate. Prominent dilated capillaries are present in the dermal papillae.

action undoubtedly plays a part. It is possible also that the vasoconstriction induced by steroids contributes to their therapeutic role in this condition.

The clinical relevance of the *vasoconstrictive effect* of topical steroids is obscure: it forms part of the anti-inflammatory actions and may contribute to the action of topical steroids in psoriasis. The vasoconstriction certainly accounts for the temporary improvement in appearance when a potent steroid is applied to the face in rosacea or 'steroid face'. It is also relevant to consider some of the side-effects of topical steroids with reference to their mechanism of action. Thinning of the skin is a reflection of their catabolic effect on skin fibroblasts and the masking of inflammation is a direct result of their anti-inflammatory properties.

REFERENCES

Balow J.E. & Rosenthal A.S. (1973). Glucocorticoid suppression of macrophage migration inhibitory factor. *J Exp Med* **137**: 1031.

Blackwell G.J., Flower R.J., Nijkamp F.P. & Vane J.R. (1978). Phospholipase A_2 activity of guinea-pig isolated perfused lungs: stimulation, and inhibition by anti-inflammatory steroids. *Br J Pharmacol* **62**: 79.

Blackwell G.J., Carnuccio R., Di Rosa M., Flower R.J., Langham C.S.J., Parente L., Persico P., Russell-Smith N.C. & Stone D. (1982). Glucocorticoids induce the formation and release of anti-inflammatory and anti-phospholipase proteins into the peritoneal cavity of the rat. *Br J Pharmacol* **76**: 185.

Burrows W.M. & Stoughton R.B. (1976). Inhibition of induction of human contact sensitization by topical glucocorticosteroids. *Arch Dermatol* **112**: 175.

Claman H.N. (1972). Corticosteroids and lymphoid cells. *N Engl J Med* **287**: 388.

Epstein E.H. & Bonifas J.M. (1982). Glucocorticoid receptors of normal human epidermis. *J Invest Dermatol* **78**: 144.

Gorski J. & Gannon F. (1976). Current models of steroid hormone action: a critique. *Annu Rev Physiol* **38**: 425.

Hammarström S., Hamberg M., Duell E.A., Stawiski M.A., Anderson T.F. & Voorhees J.J. (1977). Glucocorticoid in inflammatory proliferative skin disease reduces arachidonic and hydroxyeicosatetraenoic acids. *Science* **197**: 994.

Parrillo J.E. & Fauci A.S. (1979). Mechanisms of glucocorticoid action on immune processes. *Annu Rev Pharmacol Toxicol* **19**: 179.

Chapter 4
Potency Groups of Steroids

There is now a vast range of different compounds and formulations from which to choose when prescribing a topical steroid: over 150 such preparations are currently listed in the British National Formulary. The division of the topical steroids into four potency groups, each with its own implications for therapeutic efficacy and propensity to produce side-effects, provides a helpful guide in deciding which preparation to prescribe. It is important to understand the clinical relevance of the potency groupings and to have a thorough working knowledge of a few preparations from each group. The major topical steroids and their relevant potency groups are shown in Table 4.1.

Various methods are available for assessing the potency of topical steroids. The most widely used is the vasoconstrictor method of McKenzie & Stoughton (1962) in which corticosteroids are applied to the flexor aspect of the forearm and the intensity of the blanching effect produced is recorded. The more potent the steroid, the more intense the blanching. For example, using this method, fluocinolone acetonide is found to be 100 times more potent than hydrocortisone acetate, and betamethasone 17-valerate 3.6 times more potent than fluocinolone acetonide. Although the relevance of the vasoconstricting action of topical steroids to their therapeutic effect in skin disorders is obscure, in general, the degree of therapeutic efficacy of the steroid is in accordance with the potency as measured by the vasoconstrictor method. Other methods for assessing potency utilise the anti-mitotic and anti-inflammatory properties of cortico-

Table 4.1 The potency groups of topical steroids

Potency group	Approved name	Proprietary name
Mildly potent	hydrocortisone base or acetate 0.5%–2.5%	Efcortelan 0.5%, 1%, 2.5% Hydrocortistab 1%
Moderately potent	clobetasone butyrate 0.05% fluocinolone acetonide 0.01% flurandrenolone 0.0125% hydrocortisone 1% with urea	Eumovate Synandone Haelan Alphaderm Calmurid HC
Potent	beclomethasone dipropionate 0.025% betamethasone valerate 0.1% fluocinolone acetonide 0.025% fluocinonide 0.05% hydrocortisone butyrate 0.1% triamcinolone acetonide 0.1%	Propaderm Betnovate Synalar Metosyn Locoid Adcortyl
Very potent	beclomethasone dipropionate 0.5% clobetasol propionate 0.05% fluocinolone acetonide 0.2% diflucortolone valerate 0.3% halcinonide 0.1%	Propaderm Forte Dermovate Synalar Forte Nerisone Forte Halciderm

steroids and include, in animals, the suppression of DNA synthesis induced by application of steroids to hairless mouse skin (du Vivier & Stoughton 1975; Otani, Gange & Walter 1980) and, in humans, the measurement of degrees of suppression of experimentally induced dermatitis (Kaidbey & Kligman 1974). Potency ratings produced by these methods are comparable to those obtained in vasoconstrictor tests.

Safe and effective treatment with topical steroids depends upon knowing when to prescribe them and which potency is required (Table 4.2). The clinical relevance of the potency groups may be considered under two headings: therapeutic efficacy and unwanted effects. These major aspects of topical steroid therapy will constitute the bulk of the

Table 4.2 Choice of steroid potency

Skin disorder	Potency group
Eczema of face, flexures and in children	Mild
Eczema of trunk and limbs in adults	Moderate or Potent
Eczema of palms and soles	Potent or Very potent
Psoriasis of face and flexures	Moderate or Potent
Psoriasis of other sites Lichen simplex Lichen planus Discoid eczema Discoid lupus erythematosus Alopecia areata	Potent or Very potent

remainder of this book but it is useful in this chapter to describe the broad, general principles of the potency groups and their clinical relevance.

It is important to appreciate that the topical steroids constitute a wide range of products with vastly differing effects. The mildly potent (hydrocortisone) preparations are safe for all ages and all parts of the body and only produce adverse effects if inappropriately prescribed for a condition in which steroid therapy is contraindicated. However, hydrocortisone is ineffective in certain diseases (such as psoriasis) and in sites where the skin is thickened (such as the palms and soles or areas of lichenification). Two provisos should be added to the statement that hydrocortisone preparations are free from side-effects. Preparations which contain urea in addition to the hydrocortisone (*viz.* Calmurid HC, Alphaderm) should be placed in the moderately potent group since the urea enhances the absorption of the hydrocortisone. Secondly, hydrocortisone butyrate (Locoid), despite its name, is in fact a potent steroid. Esterification of the hydrocortisone molecule at the 17 position produces a compound which is considerably more effective than hydrocortisone and which falls into the same potency group as betamethasone valerate 0.1%.

The moderately potent topical steroids do not produce side-effects unless used indiscriminately. They are more effective than hydrocortisone but still produce no therapeutic benefit in some conditions, such as lichen planus.

Both the therapeutic efficacy and the incidence of side-effects increase sharply with the potent topical steroids. The use of these on the face, in the flexures or in children is to be discouraged and must be monitored carefully if it is absolutely necessary. They are, however, highly effective in all steroid-responsive disorders.

The very potent steroids are, of course, the most effective. The use of these agents must be carefully supervised since troublesome local side-effects are common and, if sufficient quantities are applied, absorption of the steroid will cause hypothalamic–pituitary–adrenal axis suppression.

The potency of topical steroids can be further enhanced by increasing percutaneous absorption. This can be achieved by using ointments rather than creams, lotions or gels; by adding compounds such as urea, salicylic acid or propylene glycol to increase penetration through the stratum corneum, and by occlusion with polythene, bandages or opposed skin (as in flexural sites). The amount of steroid absorbed is also significantly increased when large areas of inflamed skin are being treated.

REFERENCES

du Vivier A., Marshall R. & Brookes L. (1978). An animal model for evaluating the local and systemic effects of topically applied corticosteroids on epidermal DNA synthesis. *Br J Dermatol* **98**: 209.

du Vivier A. & Stoughton R.B. (1975). An animal model for screening topical and systemic drugs for potential use in the treatment of psoriasis. *J Invest Dermatol* **65**: 235.

Kaidbey K.H. & Kligman A.M. (1974). Assessment of topical corticosteroids by suppression of experimental inflammation in humans. *J Invest Dermatol* **63**: 292.

McKenzie A.W. & Stoughton R.B. (1962). Method for comparing percutaneous absorption of steroids. *Arch Dermatol* **86**: 608.

Otani A., Gange R. & Walter J. (1980). Epidermal DNA synthesis: a new disc technique for evaluating incorporation of tritiated thymidine. *J Invest Dermatol* **75**: 375.

STEROID POTENCY

Hydrocortisone
- Safe, even on face and in children
- Effective in eczema
- Ineffective in psoriasis
- Ineffective on thickened areas of skin

Potent steroids
- Avoid the face, flexures and children
- Monitor quantities used
- Systemic side-effects can occur

Absorption and potency increased
- By formulation
- By occlusion
- In widespread inflammatory dermatoses

Chapter 5
Correct Use As Determined By Site and Age

Successful topical corticosteroid therapy depends upon choosing a steroid of sufficient potency to be effective for the condition and site being treated but not so potent as to cause undesirable effects. Hence the site affected, the age of the patient and the disease to be treated must all be taken into consideration when deciding which steroid to prescribe.

It has been shown that there are distinct regional variations in the percutaneous absorption of compounds applied to the skin (Cronin & Stoughton 1962). These regional variations are determined by a number of factors, probably the most important being the thickness of the stratum corneum, the density of hair follicles and the richness of the vasculature in the region. Percutaneous absorption is high from the face (Fig. 5.1) and the scrotum, but low from the palms and soles (Fig. 5.2), with other regions occupying an intermediate position (Fig. 5.3). Hydration of the skin, such as occurs in flexural areas and with occlusive clothes or dressings, further increases absorption. It must not be forgotten, either, that absorption through diseased skin in which the blood supply is increased and the epidermal barrier damaged, is considerably greater than that through normal skin.

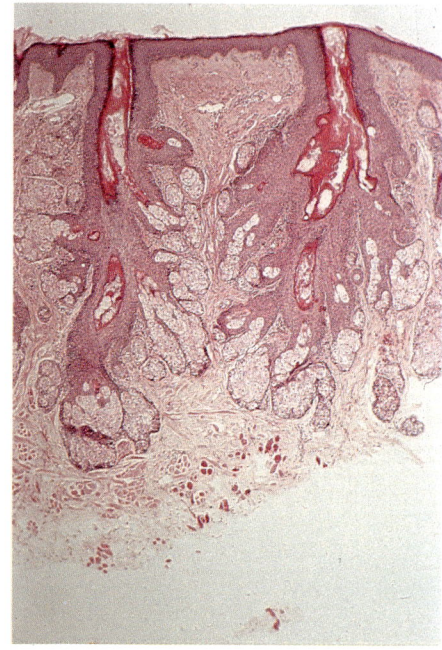

Fig. 5.1 In the normal facial skin (H & E × 15 approx.) the epidermis is thin and there are numerous pilosebaceous units, features which encourage percutaneous absorption.

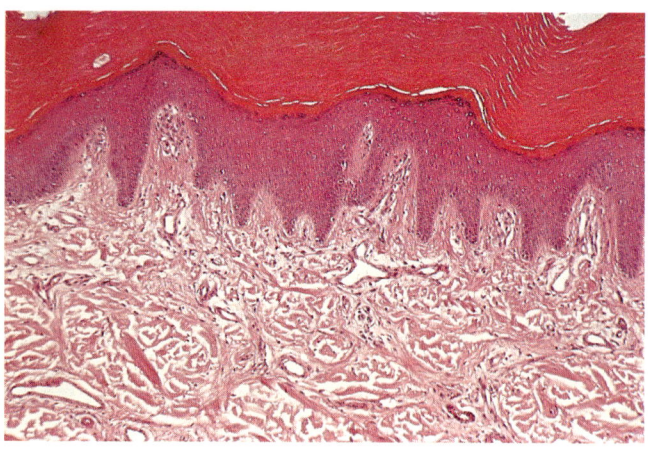

Fig. 5.2 The epidermis of the normal plantar skin (H & E × 30 approx.) is very thick with a prominent stratum corneum: percutaneous absorption is low at such sites.

SITE

Face

The face is particularly sensitive to the effects of topical steroids; percutaneous absorption is high

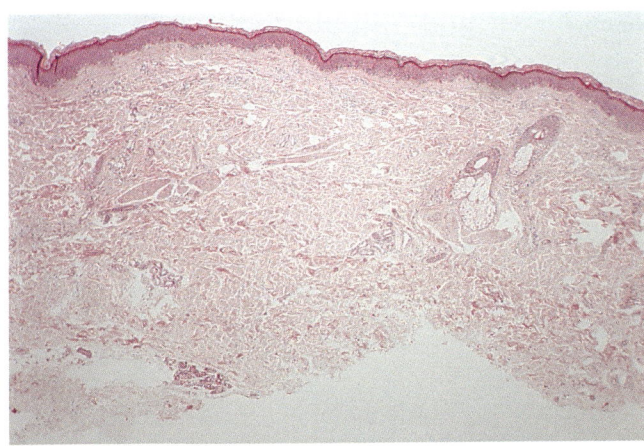

Fig. 5.3 The epidermis of the normal forearm skin (H & E × 15 approx.) is rather thin and the dermis contains occasional eccrine glands and pilosebaceous units: percutaneous absorption is intermediate between that through facial and plantar skin.

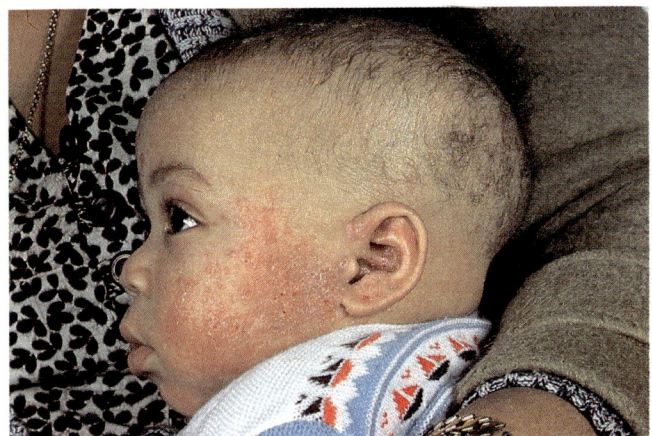

Fig. 5.4 Atopic eczema. A weak steroid such as hydrocortisone is the treatment of choice.

and adverse effects occur which are peculiar to this region (Chapter 7). The hydrocortisone preparations are safe, although even they may precipitate or worsen acne vulgaris in susceptible individuals. It should be possible to manage most cases of facial eczema (Fig. 5.4) with a hydrocortisone preparation but an acute or severe eczema, together with many cases of psoriasis and all the other less common steroid-responsive disorders will require treatment with a more potent topical steroid (Fig. 5.5). This should be for as short a time as possible: one or two

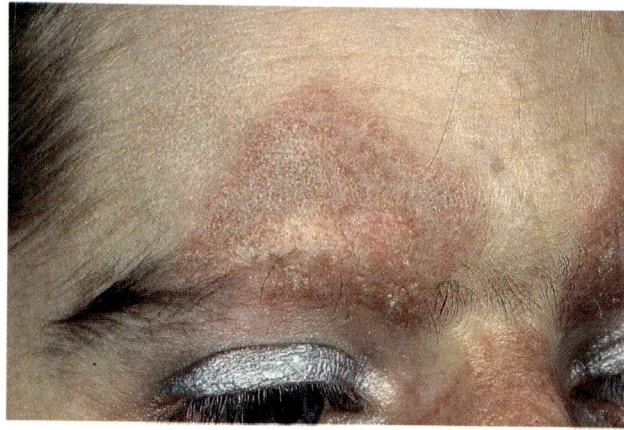

Fig. 5.5 Discoid lupus erythematosus. A potent steroid will be required.

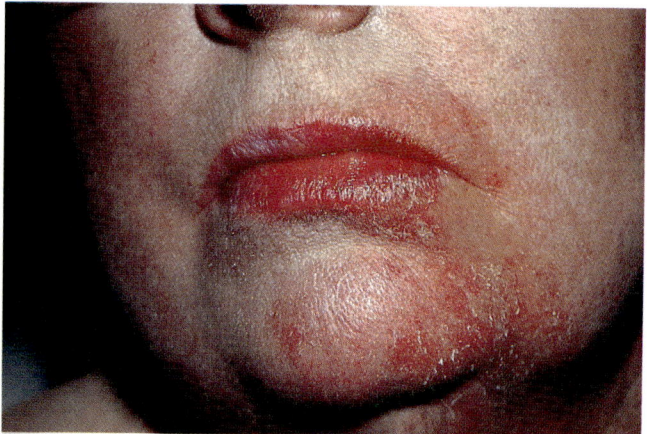

Fig. 5.6 Contact dermatitis to nail varnish. This facial eczema failed to clear with topical steroids until the allergen was identified by patch testing and the patient stopped using nail varnish.

weeks at the most of daily applications. Thereafter the treatment of eczema should be maintained with a less potent steroid while other conditions may be kept under control using short, intermittent courses of a potent preparation. The amount of steroid used by the patient should be monitored carefully and the face examined regularly for evidence of side-effects.

If the rash does not respond to steroid treatment (Fig. 5.6), it is important to consider whether a **contact allergy** may be perpetuating the eruption (e.g. to cosmetics or nail varnish) or if the diagnosis is correct: is it in fact **acne or rosacea**?

Flexures and genitalia

The very nature of these sites makes occlusion, and hence increased effects of the topical steroids, unavoidable. In addition the thin skin of the male genitalia, in particular the scrotum, further enhances these effects. Atrophy of the skin with striae is readily produced if potent steroids are applied to these sites (Fig. 5.7). Hydrocortisone preparations are safe and should be used whenever possible.

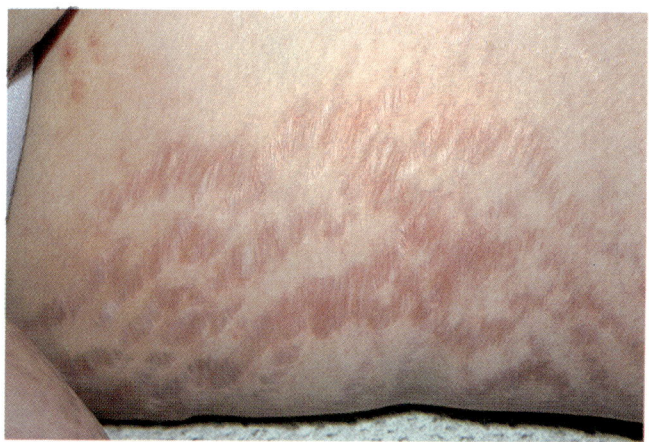

Fig. 5.7 Inguinal striae. Prolonged application of excessive quantities of potent topical steroids in this occluded site was responsible.

However, severe eczemas and many cases of psoriasis will not respond and a moderately potent or potent steroid will be required. Intermittent courses of treatment with these preparations are preferable to continuous long-term applications.

If response to treatment is poor, consider whether the diagnosis is correct: is it in fact an infection, e.g. **candida, tinea or erythrasma**?

Scalp

The scalp is relatively spared from the side-effects of topical steroids because of the thickness of the

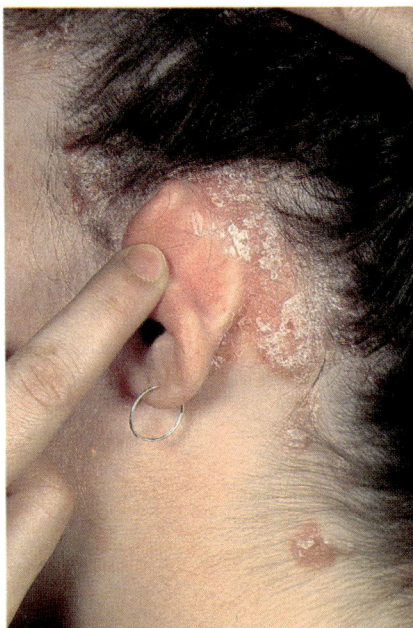

Fig. 5.8 Scalp psoriasis. A potent steroid will be required usually in conjunction with tar and a keratolytic agent.

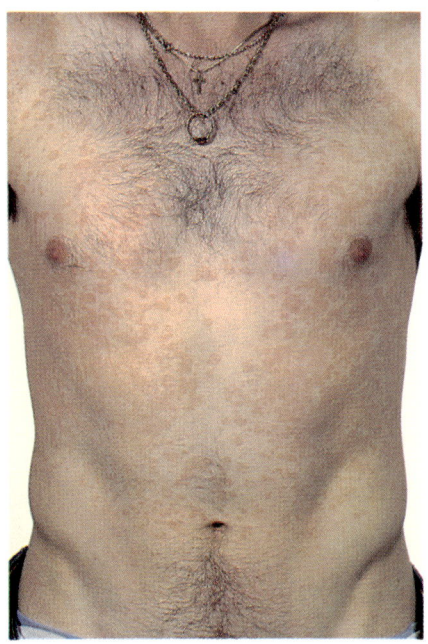

Fig. 5.9 Pityriasis versicolor. Extensive involvement like this has usually been misdiagnosed as eczema or pityriasis rosea and treated inappropriately with a topical steroid.

stratum corneum. In general, hydrocortisone preparations are ineffective and more potent steroids are required (Fig. 5.8).

If the condition does not respond consider whether the diagnosis is correct: could it be **solar keratoses** on a bald scalp and not eczema at all?

Trunk

The decision on steroid potency for the trunk depends upon the disease being treated (*see* Chapter 6) and the age of the patient. Any steroid applied to the back or presternal area may precipitate or worsen acne but otherwise there are no particular contraindications to the use of potent steroids on

Correct Use as Determined by Site and Age   27

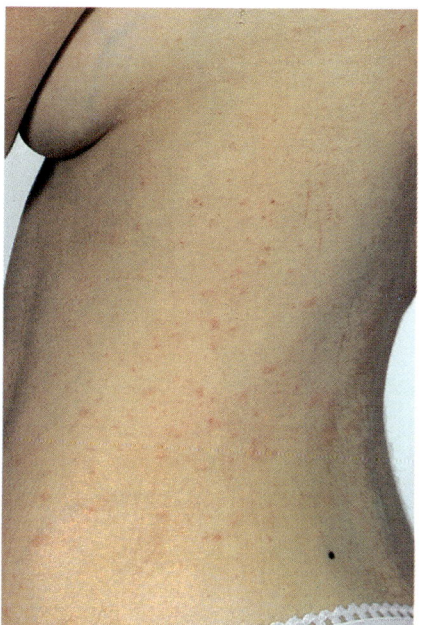

Fig. 5.10 Scabies. The presence of an itchy papular eruption on the trunk should prompt examination of the hands and feet for burrows and of the genitalia for papules and nodules.

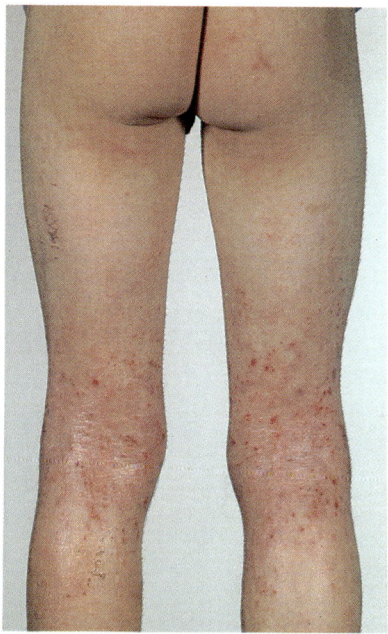

Fig. 5.11 Atopic eczema. A potent steroid will be required to clear this degree of eczema in an adult. Any maintenance treatment should be with the weakest possible steroid.

the trunk beyond the usual precaution of using the preparation sparingly.

If the eruption does not improve, consider whether the diagnosis is correct: **pityriasis versicolor** (Fig. 5.9), **acne vulgaris** and **scabies** (Fig. 5.10) are examples of common, non-steroid-responsive conditions affecting the trunk.

Limbs

As for the trunk, the decision on steroid potency rests more with the disease being treated and the age of the patient than with the site. In an adult, hydrocortisone preparations are rarely effective (Fig. 5.11) except for treating mild eczema. Potent steroids may produce a folliculitis on the limbs and, if treatment is continued long term, striae may develop, usually affecting the inner aspects of the upper arms and thighs. Particular mention should be made of the lower leg with varicose eczema. Potent steroids used in this situation will further thin the already compromised skin and encourage incipient ulceration (*see* p. 36).

If response to treatment is unsatisfactory, consider whether there is an element of **folliculitis** requiring the addition of a systemic antibiotic. If the condition being treated is a varicose eczema, consider whether the patient has developed a **contact allergy** to one of the constituents of the treatment being used, e.g. antibiotic or preservative in a cream.

Hands and feet

The palms and soles form a separate category for here the stratum corneum is so thick that only the potent steroids will penetrate sufficiently to produce any beneficial therapeutic effect. In fact it is frequently necessary to use steroids from the very potent group together with polythene occlusion to treat eczema or psoriasis of the palms and soles. Side-effects do not often occur at these sites but should, of course, be looked for regularly. The difference between the skin of the palms and soles and that of the rest of the body (especially the dorsa of the hands and feet) should be pointed out to the patient so that he takes special care not to allow the steroid to spread from the palms and soles. Prolonged solar damage renders the dorsa of the hands particularly sensitive to the effects of potent steroids and purpura and atrophy develop readily (Fig 5.12).

If response to treatment is inadequate consider whether other factors are at work and need attention, e.g. infection, either due to **tinea** or **secondary bacterial invasion**, or **contact dermatitis**, either allergic or primary irritant.

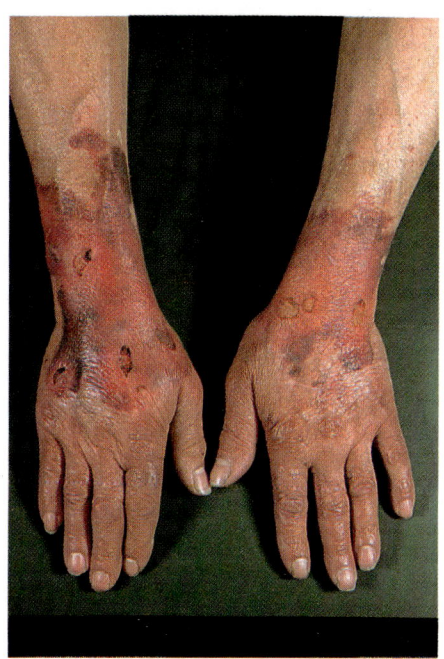

Fig. 5.12 Steroid-induced atrophy. Marked atrophy with erythema, purpura and erosions have been produced by prolonged application of excessive quantities of a very potent steroid.

AGE

Children

Adverse systemic effects in the form of hypothalamic-pituitary-adrenal axis suppression with resultant growth retardation occur more readily in children than in adults (Feiwel 1969; Feiwel, James & Barnett 1969). This is because of the increased ratio of surface area to volume in children and is a particular danger in infants. Topical steroids other than hydrocortisone should, therefore, be used with great caution in children and should rarely be prescribed for infants.

The main indications for using topical steroids in children are atopic eczema, seborrhoeic eczema and primary irritant napkin dermatitis. A hydrocortisone preparation should be adequate for most cases provided other aspects of therapy such as removing irritants and treating itch, infection, and dry skin are managed appropriately. Eczema of the trunk and limbs which is acute, severe, lichenified or discoid may require a stronger steroid. The use of potent steroids in the napkin area should be avoided in view of the risk of producing infantile gluteal granulomata (Chapter 7).

Psoriasis in children should, if possible, be managed without the use of topical steroids although short courses may be necessary for flexural psoriasis.

Old age

The dermis becomes thinned in old age. As a result of prolonged solar damage and age-related degenerative changes, the amount of collagen decreases and the elastin becomes fragmented. Application of potent topical steroids will exacerbate this change and the side-effects of the steroids such as atrophy, purpura and telangiectasia will occur more readily. In addition, there is evidence that drugs are cleared from the skin more slowly in the elderly with consequent potentiation of their effects. Prolonged use of potent topical steroids in the elderly should therefore be avoided wherever possible.

REFERENCES

Cronin E. & Stoughton R.B. (1962). Percutaneous absorption: regional variations and the effect of hydration and epidermal stripping. *Br J Dermatol* **74**: 265.

Feiwel M. (1969). Percutaneous absorption of topical steroids in children. *Br J Dermatol* **81**(4): 113.

Feiwel M., James V.H.T. & Barnett E.S. (1969). Effect of potent topical steroids on plasma cortisol levels of infants and children with eczema. *Lancet* **i**: 485.

REGIONAL FACTORS IN PERCUTANEOUS ABSORPTION

- Thickness of stratum corneum
- Degree of erythema
- Density of hair follicles
- Hydration of skin

SITE

Face
- Use hydrocortisone whenever possible

Flexures
- Use hydrocortisone but short courses of a more potent steroid may be necessary

Palms and soles
- Need potent steroids

AGE

Children
- Beware systemic effects
- Use hydrocortisone whenever possible

Old age
- Beware the lower leg
- Local side-effects occur readily

Chapter 6
Correct Use As Determined By Disease

ECZEMA

The terms eczema and dermatitis are synonymous and embrace a wide range of clinical pictures, all characterised by inflammation of the skin. Eczema affects people of all ages and can involve any part of the body. In order to establish certain guidelines it is helpful to classify eczema into its accepted forms.

Endogenous eczemas

Atopic eczema

Atopic eczema is common, occurring primarily in children (Figs 6.1, 6.2) but occasionally persisting into adult life. Two important facets of atopic eczema dictate caution in the use of topical steroids: the young age of the majority of the patients and the chronicity of the disease. The aim of treatment

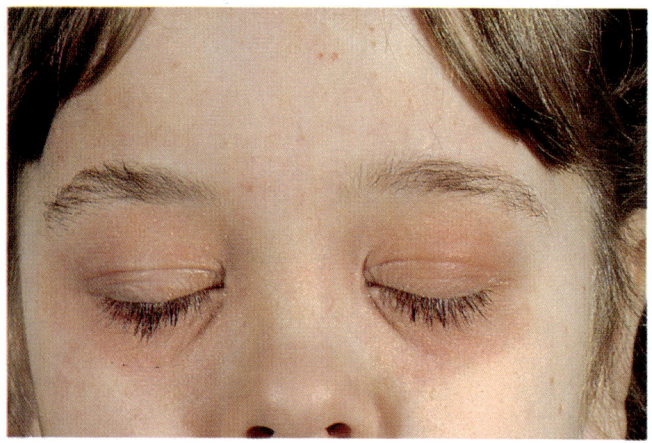

Fig. 6.1 Atopic eczema. Involvement of the eyelids is characteristic and should be treated with a hydrocortisone preparation only.

Correct Use as Determined by Disease 33

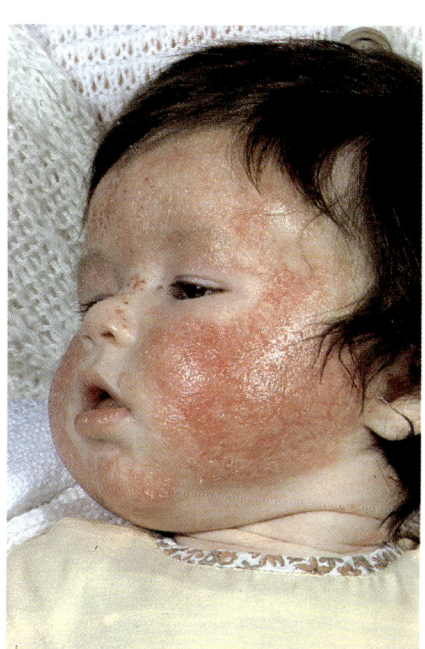

Fig. 6.2 Atopic eczema. The face is usually involved in infantile atopic eczema. Steroids of mild potency only should be used.

should be to control the disease long term with the weakest possible topical steroid, preferably 1% hydrocortisone. Effective management of other aspects of the disease such as pruritus, dry skin and infection will often help to achieve this aim. A steroid from the moderately potent group is often required to control atopic eczema of the trunk and limbs in an adult and in severe, lichenified childhood eczema (Fig. 6.3). Acute exacerbations may be treated with a potent steroid but this should be short term and the amount used by the patient must be monitored carefully. A potent steroid is required to treat eczema of the palms and soles.

Secondary infection with staphylococci is common in atopic eczema (Fig. 6.4), particularly in children and is often the cause of an exacerbation of the eczema and failure to respond to topical steroids. In such situations systemic antibiotics are necessary. When recurrent infection is a problem, long-term,

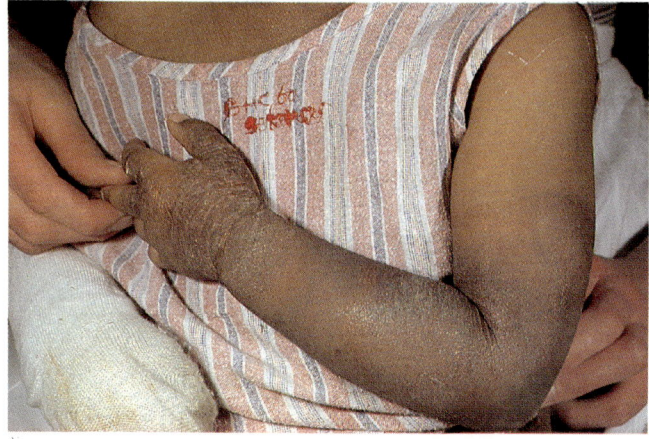

Fig. 6.3 Atopic eczema. Chronic, lichenified eczema on the limbs may require a moderately potent steroid for a short time. Emollients, antihistamines and occlusive bandaging are also helpful.

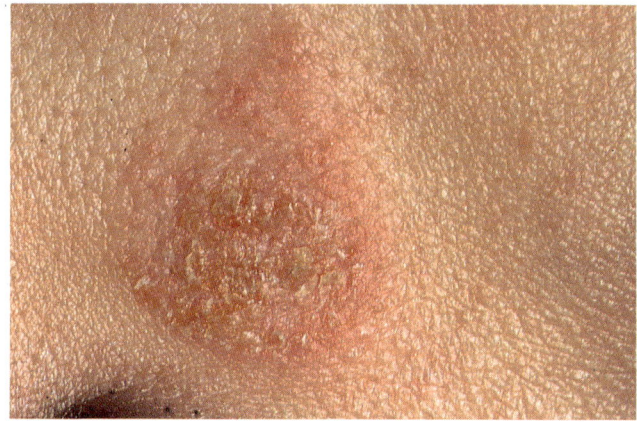

Fig. 6.4 Impetiginised eczema. The golden exudate indicates secondary infection. A systemic antibiotic is necessary in this situation.

low-dose antibiotic therapy or the use of a combined anti-infective steroid preparation may prevent relapses due to infection, provide better control of the eczema and obviate the need for stronger steroids.

It is important to also remember that viral infections do occur in atopic subjects and may be mistaken by the patient for the lesions of eczema. Mollusca contagiosa, warts and herpes simplex infections will spread if treated inappropriately with topical steroids.

Seborrhoeic eczema

Seborrhoeic eczema is a variant of eczema which

occurs most often in young adults and involves the central portions of the face (Fig. 6.5), chest and back, the scalp and the major flexures (Fig. 6.6). The facial eruption will respond to a hydrocortisone preparation but a stronger steroid is required for other sites, together with a tar shampoo. If a potent steroid

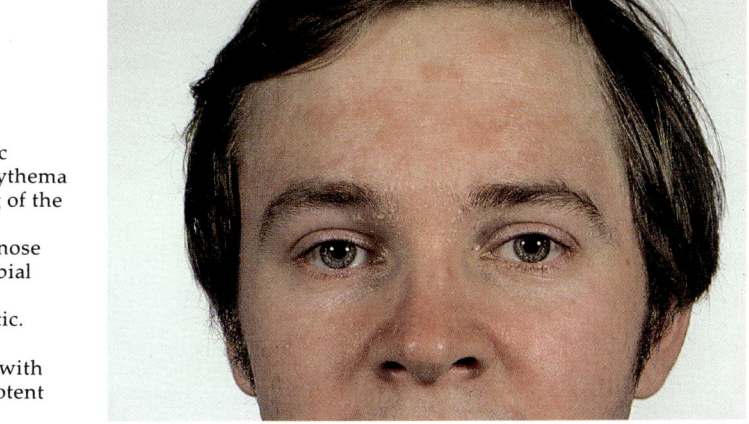

Fig. 6.5 Seborrhoeic eczema. Erythema and scaling of the forehead, eyebrows, nose and nasolabial folds is characteristic. Treatment should be with a mildly potent steroid.

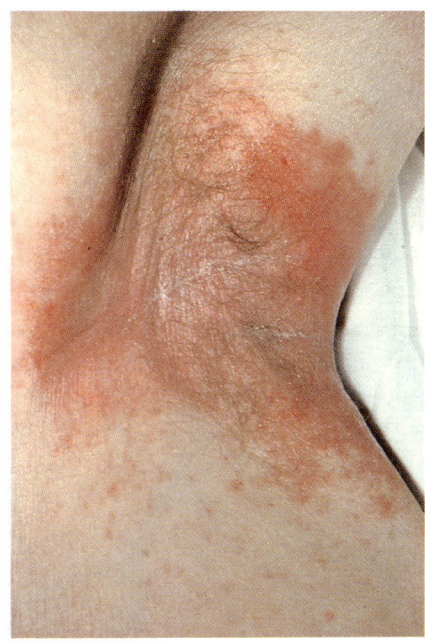

Fig. 6.6 Seborrhoeic eczema. The axilla is another common site for this condition. Prolonged use of potent steroids should be avoided at this site because of the risk of side-effects.

is necessary to control seborrhoeic eczema in the inguinal region, it is important to advise the patient to use the treatment sparingly and, if possible, in short, intermittent courses because of the risk of producing atrophy and striae at this site.

Seborrhoeic eczema of infancy

This is a common condition in which erythema and a characterstic yellow scaling affects mainly the face, scalp and the major flexures. Sometimes the whole body is involved. Treatment is with emollients and a hydrocortisone preparation. Secondary infection is common, especially in the napkin area, when a combined anti-infective steroid preparation is required.

Varicose eczema

Chronic venous insufficiency in the leg produces varicosities, oedema, purpura, brown pigmentation of the skin due to haemosiderin deposition, eczema and, ultimately, ulceration (Fig. 6.7). A potent steroid may be required initially to control the eczema but maintenance treatment should be with the weakest effective preparation and the steroid must not be applied to areas of ulceration. Patients with varicose eczema readily develop contact allergies and so creams, which contain sensitising preservatives, and topical antibiotics or combined anti-infective steroid preparations should not be used. Measures directed at controlling the underlying pathology are an important part of management: varicose veins should be treated when possible, elastic stockings must be worn and patients advised on the use of emollients and on elevation and exercise of the legs.

Discoid eczema

Discoid eczema, even in children, rarely responds to

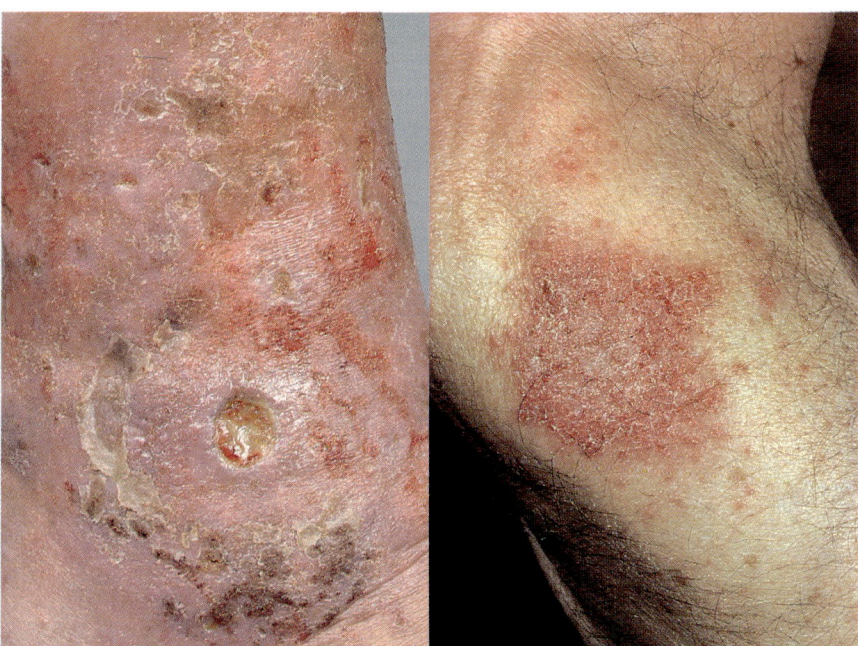

Fig. 6.7 Varicose eczema with ulceration. A steroid may be necessary to treat the eczema but should not be applied to the area of ulceration.

Fig. 6.8 Discoid eczema. A potent steroid is usually necessary and it is important to treat secondary infection which is common in this condition.

the weaker topical steroids. A steroid from the potent group is usually required and this is safe provided that the patient applies small amounts to the affected areas only. Discoid eczema on the limbs of an adult (Fig. 6.8) may require a very potent steroid but this should be for as short a time as possible. Secondary infection is common in discoid eczema and a course of oral antibiotics or a combined antibiotic-steroid topical preparation is often required to achieve adequate control.

Pompholyx

Since pompholyx affects the palms and soles (Fig. 6.9), it requires a potent or very potent topical steroid. Other aspects of management such as potassium permanganate or aluminium acetate soaks and oral antibiotics if required must be used.

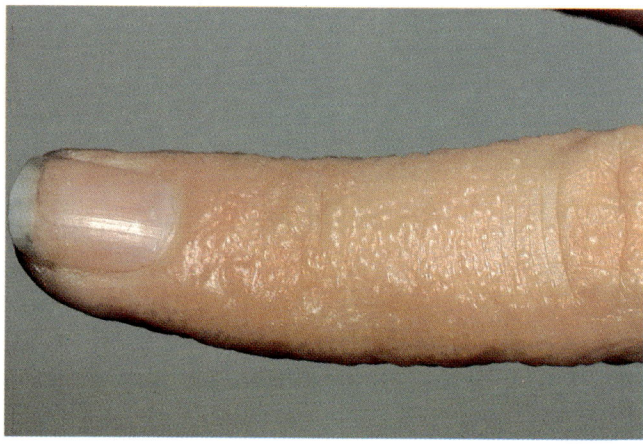

Fig. 6.9 Pompholyx. A potent steroid is required. Aluminium acetate soaks and systemic antihistamines will ease the intense itching.

Exogenous eczemas

Primary irritant eczema

Primary irritant eczema occurs in skin which has been exposed to physical or chemical irritants. Detergents and water are the commonest irritants. The type of primary irritant eczema seen most frequently is the hand eczema affecting housewives, mothers and those people who often have their hands in soapy water (Fig. 6.10). Many such patients probably have an underlying atopic tendency predisposing their skin to react to irritants. In the initial stages of treatment a potent topical steroid will usually be necessary to control the inflammation, but liberal use of emollients and advice on avoiding irritants are vital in the long-term management.

Correct Use as Determined by Disease 39

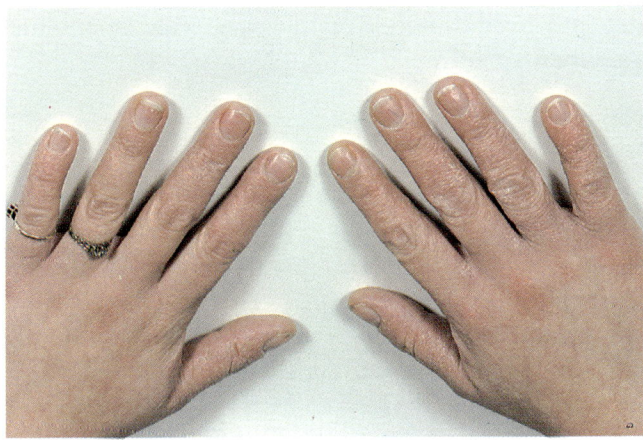

Fig. 6.10 Primary irritant eczema. Advice on protecting the hands from irritants and on the use of emollients is of more value than steroid therapy.

Asteatotic eczema (eczema craquelé) is another type of primary irritant eczema in which the skin becomes excessively dry (Fig. 6.11). It is common in the elderly, because their skin becomes intolerant to the drying effect of ordinary washing with soap and water, and in hospital inpatients as a result of bed

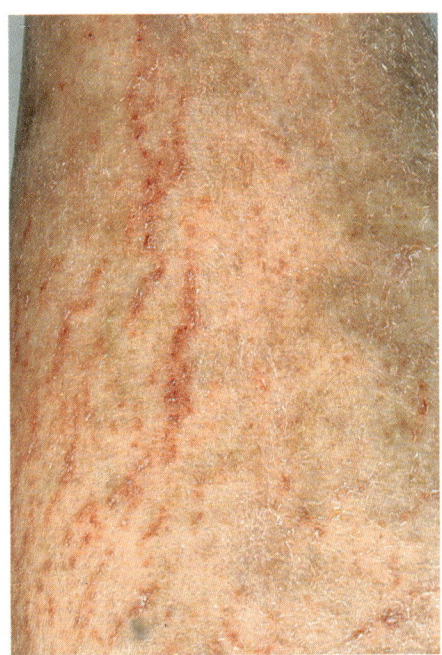

Fig. 6.11 Eczema craquelé. The tramline cracking of the skin is characteristic. This is common in the elderly and responds to emollients rather than to topical steroids.

baths in the hospital environment which is usually dry and over-heated. Treatment is with emollients and soap substitutes.

Napkin dermatitis

This is a type of irritant eczema produced by urine and faeces in prolonged contact with the skin in an occluded environment (Fig. 6.12). Tight disposable nappies and plastic pants predispose to the development of napkin dermatitis. The rash is worst in areas directly in contact with the nappy and the crevices of the creases are usually spared. The mother must be advised to leave the area exposed for as much of the time as is practicable, and she must be advised on the importance of regular nappy changes and the use of barrier creams when nappies have to be used. A soap substitute should be prescribed to reduce further the irritants contacting the skin. A hydrocortisone preparation will be required to control the inflammation and, since secondary infection with candida or bacteria is common, a combined steroid anti-infective agent is desirable. In severe cases, a moderately potent steroid may be required but this should be for as short a time as possible.

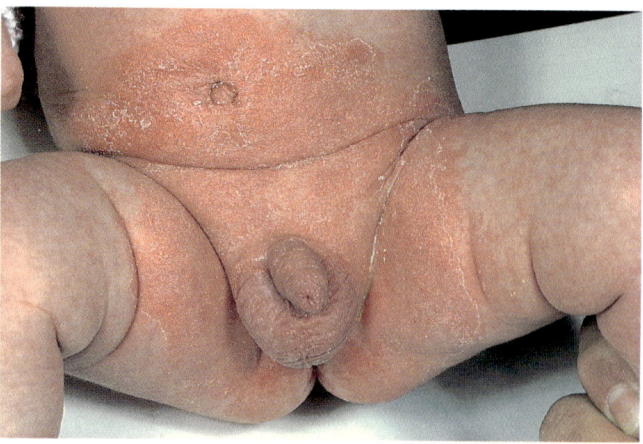

Fig. 6.12 Napkin dermatitis. This is a further type of primary irritant eczema and advice on reducing contact with the causative irritant factors must be given. A mild steroid is usually required, sometimes in combination with an anti-bacterial and anti-candidal agent.

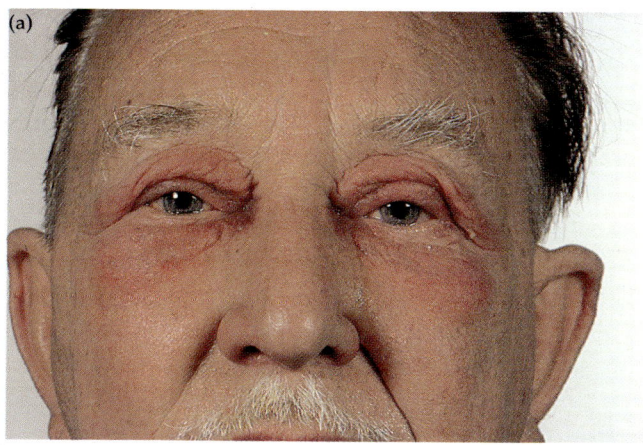

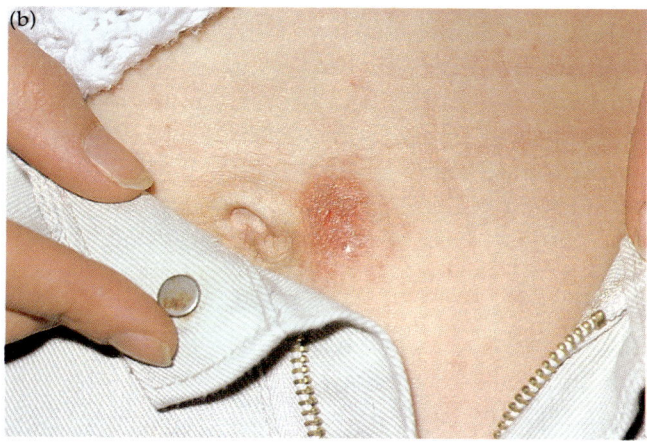

Fig. 6.13 Contact dermatitis. (a) Contact dermatitis to a topical antihistamine preparation. Acute eczema around the eyes of an adult is often the result of a contact allergy (b); contact dermatitis to nickel. The zips and studs on jeans are now a common source of this allergen.

Allergic contact eczema

Allergic contact eczema (Fig. 6.13) must be fully investigated with an adequate history of the patient's work and hobby contacts, examination of the skin and patch testing. Topical steroids will be required to control the eczema, the strength needed depending upon the site and severity of the eczema. Avoidance of the allergen is obviously important to prevent persistence or recurrence of the problem.

PSORIASIS

The place of topical steroids in the treatment of psoriasis is complex. The antimitotic and anti-inflammatory actions of the potent topical steroids certainly suppress the lesions of psoriasis but cessation of treatment often leads to a rebound worsening of the disease process. Psoriasis over-treated with very potent steroids may become unstable or even pustular which is a dangerous and occasionally fatal complication. Furthermore, psoriasis is a chronic disease requiring long-term treatment so that the development of side-effects from topical steroid therapy is more likely.

Topical steroids, therefore, are not the treatment of choice for extensive chronic plaque psoriasis: tar, dithranol and phototherapy should be used in preference. However, the majority of people with psoriasis have minor involvement of small areas of the body and in such cases intermittent courses of potent topical steroids are certainly justified, particularly since patients find them more acceptable and easier to use than the alternative messy and time-consuming treatments. The drawbacks of topical steroid therapy should be discussed with the patient who should be advised that alternative therapy will be necessary if the psoriasis becomes more extensive or resistant to the treatment being used. In general, topical steroids ameliorate psoriasis but do not produce the significant remissions from the disease which can be obtained with other modes of treatment.

Tar and dithranol, however, are too irritant to be used on the face and in the flexures and it is for psoriasis in these areas that topical steroids are definitely indicated. The weaker steroids are rarely effective and most patients will require intermittent courses of treatment with a potent steroid. Care should be taken in flexural areas (Fig. 6.14) because of the risk of producing striae. Topical steroids

Correct Use as Determined by Disease 43

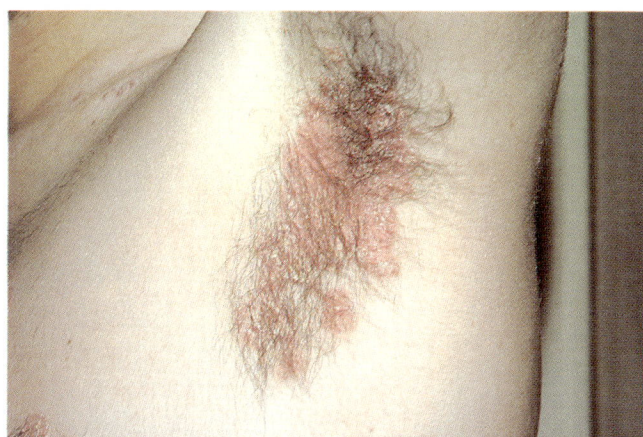

Fig. 6.14 Psoriasis of the axilla. If a moderately potent steroid is ineffective, a potent preparation may be tried.

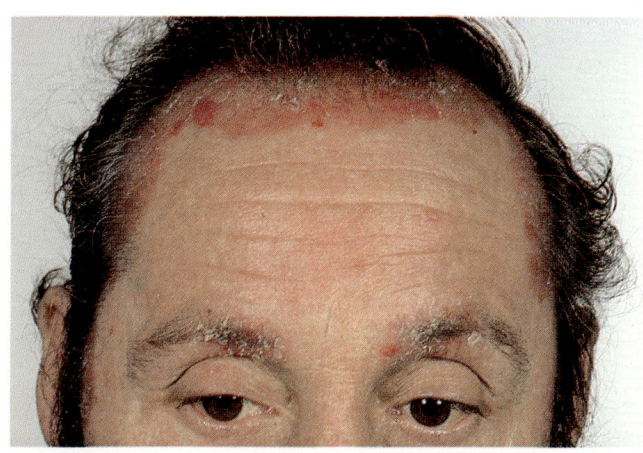

Fig. 6.15 Scalp psoriasis. A potent steroid may be necessary in conjunction with tar, dithranol or keratolytic preparations.

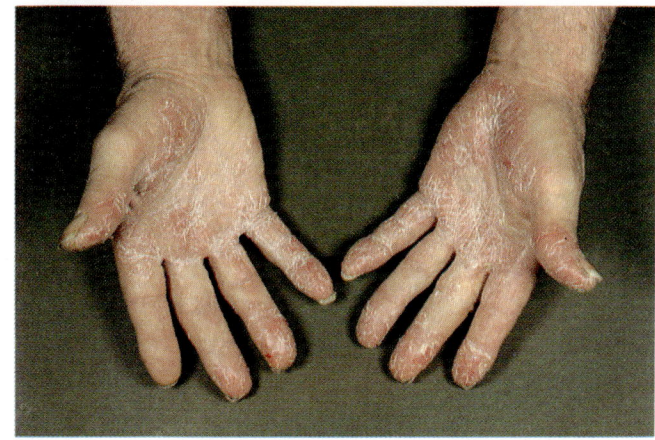

Fig. 6.16 Psoriasis of the palms. Due to the extreme thickness of the stratum corneum only very potent steroids will be effective. They should be used in conjunction with dithranol and keratolytic agents.

are also indicated for psoriasis of the scalp (Fig. 6.15) but should preferably be used in conjunction with tar, dithranol or keratolytic agents. Similarly, psoriasis of the palms (Fig. 6.16) and soles is often best controlled by potent or very potent steroids, sometimes with polythene occlusion, in conjunction with a dithranol or keratolytic preparation.

Psoriasis in childhood is best treated with tar and ultraviolet light. Topical steroids should be avoided whenever possible since the safe, mildly potent preparations are usually ineffective.

LICHEN PLANUS

This self-limiting eruption (Fig. 6.17) responds only to the stronger topical steroids and treatment with very potent preparations such as clobetasol propionate is often required to control the itching and obviate the need for systemic steroids. The amount of steroid used by the patient should be monitored. Topical steroids may also be used in the mouth to treat oral lichen planus. Regular treatment of large areas of the body is rarely necessary for more than a few weeks although persistent areas may require attention for months or even years.

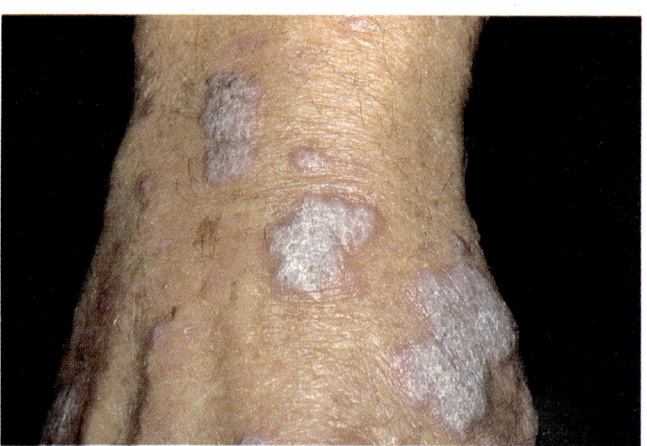

Fig. 6.17 Hypertrophic lichen planus. Weak steroids are ineffective and a very potent steroid or even intralesional triamcinolone may be required to achieve any therapeutic response.

LICHEN SIMPLEX AND NODULAR PRURIGO

The stratum corneum is greatly thickened in these conditions (Figs. 6.18, 6.19) and hence only the powerful topical steroids have any therapeutic

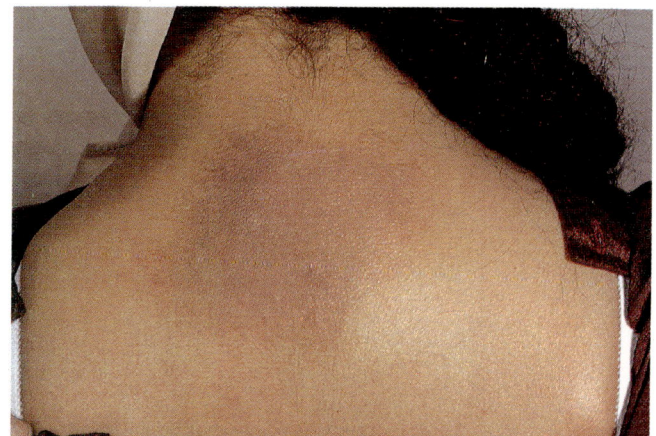

Fig. 6.18 Lichen simplex. Potent or intralesional steroids help but measures to reduce anxiety and scratching are vital in the management of this potentially chronic condition.

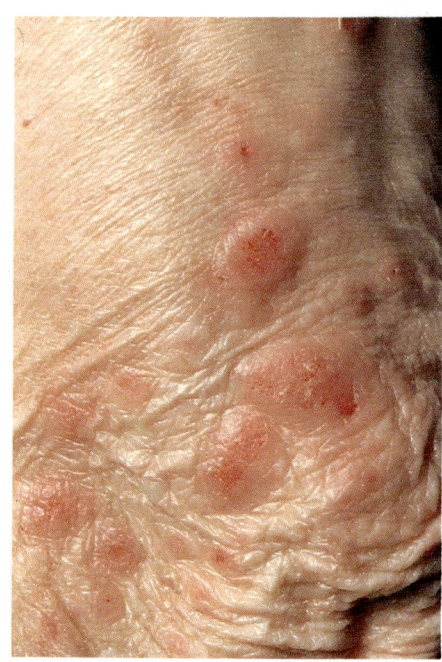

Fig. 6.19 Nodular prurigo. Treatment is very difficult but potent steroids with occlusion or intralesional steroids are usually tried.

effect. Measures such as oral antihistamines and protective bandaging must also be taken to prevent further scratching, but effective treatment is often difficult. Intralesional injections of steroids may help to suppress the itching.

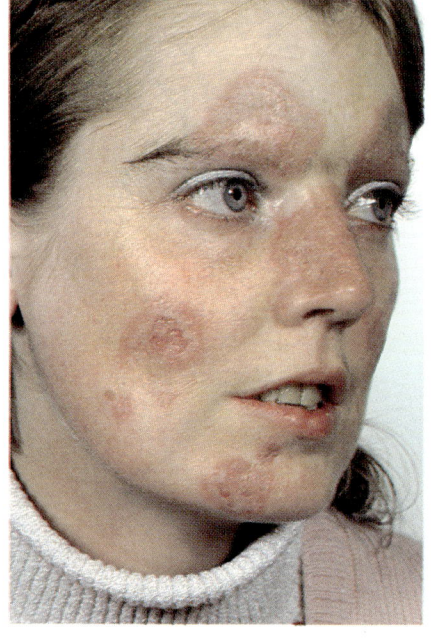

Fig. 6.20 Discoid lupus erythematosus. Only the more potent steroids are effective in this condition. Despite the site, daily application of a potent preparation to active lesions is the treatment of choice.

DISCOID LUPUS ERYTHEMATOSUS

Just as systemic steroids are effective in treating systemic lupus erythematosus, so the potent and very potent topical steroids will usually suppress any active lesions of the cutaneous variant of the disease (Fig. 6.20). Treatment should be monitored carefully and stopped when the disease appears to be inactive, particularly since the face is so commonly affected in discoid lupus erythematosus.

Correct Use as Determined by Disease 47

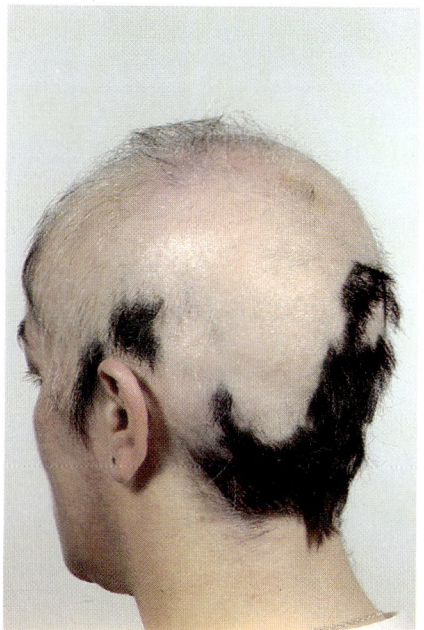

Fig. 6.21 Alopecia areata. Recovery of hair growth may be accelerated by intralesional or potent topical steroids.

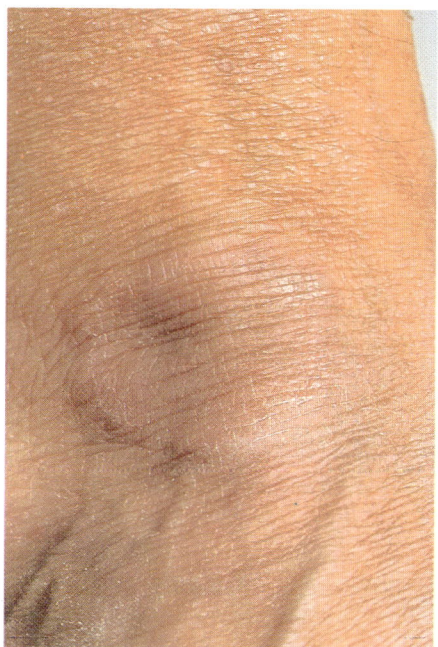

Fig. 6.22 Granuloma annulare. Intralesional steroids produce the best response.

ALOPECIA AREATA

Potent topical and intralesional steroids are frequently used in alopecia areata (Fig. 6.21). They probably hasten spontaneous resolution in active lesions but their efficacy is not fully established and over-treatment should be avoided.

GRANULOMATOUS CONDITIONS

Granuloma annulare (Fig. 6.22), necrobiosis lipoidica and sarcoidosis may be treated by potent topical steroids or by intralesional steroids. Not all cases respond, however, and over-enthusiastic treatment may produce unsightly atrophic areas so careful supervision is required.

MISCELLANEOUS CONDITIONS

Any inflammatory, non-infected lesion may respond to topical steroid therapy and a limited period of treatment can be helpful in controlling symptoms from insect bites and sunburn in particular. Intralesional steroids are often used in the treatment of keloid scars but their efficacy is limited.

ECZEMA

Atopic eczema
- Use weakest effective topical steroid
- Remember to treat: dry skin
  pruritus
  secondary infection

Discoid and pompholyx eczemas
- Potent steroid required

Hand eczema
- Remember: advice on avoiding irritants
  effective use of emollients
  is there an allergic contact factor?

Failure of treatment in eczema
- Is diagnosis correct?
- Is patch testing necessary?

ALTERNATIVE TREATMENTS FOR PSORIASIS

Topical
- Tar
- Dithranol
- Salicylic acid
- Ultraviolet B radiation

Systemic
- Methotrexate
- PUVA
- Etretinate
- Hydroxyurea

Chapter 7
Side-effects

These may be divided into the local side-effects, occurring at the sites of application of the steroid, and the systemic side-effects. All of these side-effects occur more readily and with greater frequency with increasing potency of steroid. Many of the local side-effects now seen from topical steroids are not directly attributable to the drugs themselves but to incorrect prescribing. This may be either because steroids are prescribed inappropriately to treat the wrong condition (i.e. incorrect diagnosis) or because a steroid of too great a potency has been prescribed for the condition being treated. A further cause of the misuse of steroids is incorrect use by the patient who either applies too much or uses them for the wrong purposes. It is not uncommon for patients to leave in their bathroom cabinet a tube of a potent topical steroid appropriately prescribed, e.g. for hand eczema, and then for the patient or a member of the family to start applying the steroid to treat their acne. When prescribed and used correctly, side-effects from topical steroids are uncommon.

LOCAL SIDE-EFFECTS

Atrophy of the skin

This is the most frequent complication of treatment with potent topical steroids and can produce severe cosmetic disability as well as troublesome clinical problems. One of the earliest reported side-effects of the topical steroids was the development of atrophic striae (*see* Fig. 5.7) in patients being treated for inguinal intertrigo (Epstein, Epstein & Epstein 1963). Steroids cause thinning of both the dermis and the epidermis (Kirby & Munro 1976) apparent clinically as transparency of the skin with striae, purpura and telangiectasia (Fig. 7.1). These features will appear at any site with prolonged use of potent steroids but

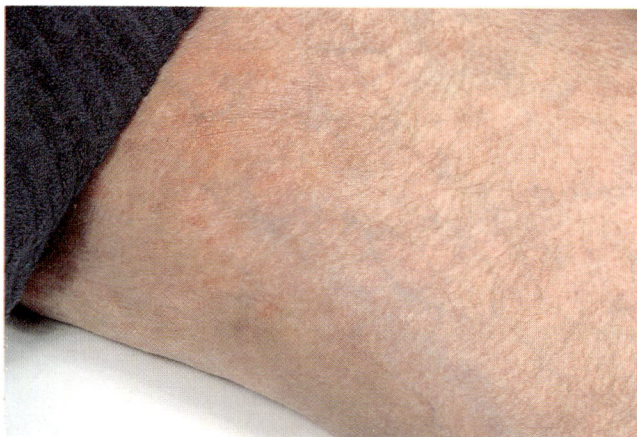

Fig. 7.1 Cutaneous atrophy. Extreme thinning of the skin and striae produced by long-term excessive use of a potent steroid for eczema.

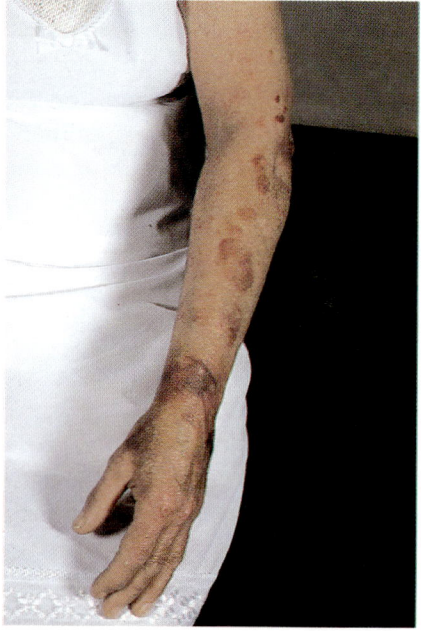

Fig. 7.2 Purpura. The result of prolonged excessive use of a potent steroid for eczema.

susceptible sites, particularly the flexures, will develop such side-effects readily, sometimes after only a few applications of a very potent preparation. However, it is not uncommon to find that, in many patients with severe flexural striae, the steroids have been inappropriately used to treat a fungal infection and not a steroid-responsive disorder.

A further result of the cutaneous atrophy produced by topical steroids is that the skin is extremely fragile. It tears and bruises easily ('steroid purpura') (Fig. 7.2) and, because steroids inhibit the formation of new collagen, healing is impaired. These features can be a particular problem if gravitational eczema is treated with potent steroids since they may produce frank ulceration and certainly prevent ulcers from healing.

Masking of infection

Corticosteroids suppress the inflammatory changes which normally accompany an infection but there is no good evidence that they actually potentiate infections. Daltrey & Cunliffe (1983) found that regular application of betamethasone 17-valerate did not alter the number of micro-organisms present. However, in flexural sites and under polythene occlusion, staphylococcal folliculitis (Fig. 7.3) and candidiasis may develop during topical steroid treatment.

It is not uncommon for topical steroids to be prescribed inappropriately for primary infective disorders of the skin. There is often an initial improvement in the eruption because of the reduction in inflammation, and hence the clinical signs of the infection are masked or altered and the infecting organism is not eradicated. Treatment of scabies with topical steroids produces a widespread crusted eruption with numerous burrows but little inflammation. Fungal infections are frequently misdiagnosed as eczema: pityriasis versicolor treated with potent steroids becomes florid and widespread

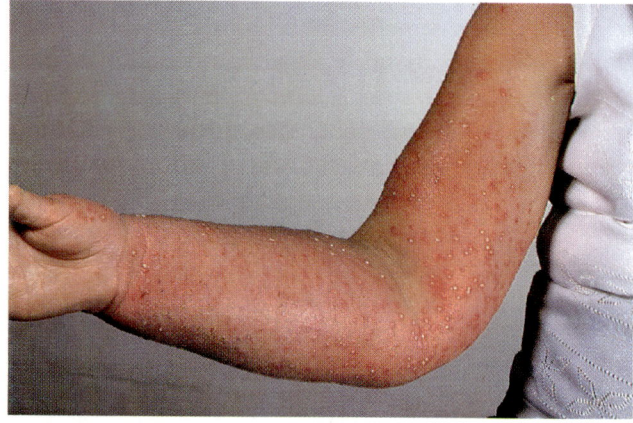

Fig. 7.3 Folliculitis. This is associated with steroid use.

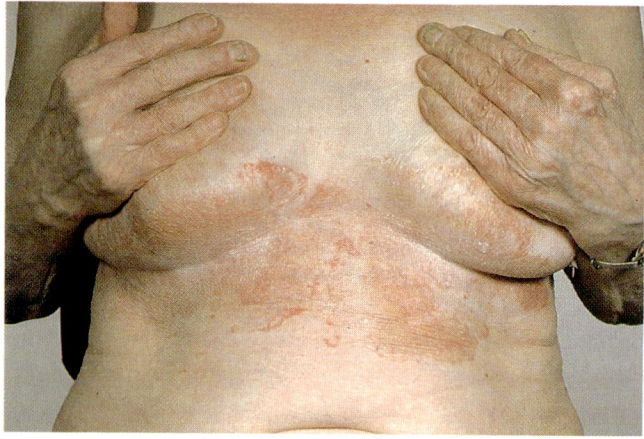

Fig. 7.4 Tinea incognito. The inflammatory response to the tinea infection has been suppressed by the steroid: the eruption has spread and the edge is not clearly defined.

while application of steroids to tinea infections produces a bizarre clinical picture known as tinea incognito (Ive & Marks 1968). In this condition the usual raised scaly margin and inflammation of a tinea infection is lost (Fig. 7.4) and the affected area shows a bruise-like discolouration with nodules and sometimes pustules at the margin (Fig. 7.5).

Steroid acne

Topical steroids worsen pre-existing acne vulgaris and can also precipitate a variant of acne. The

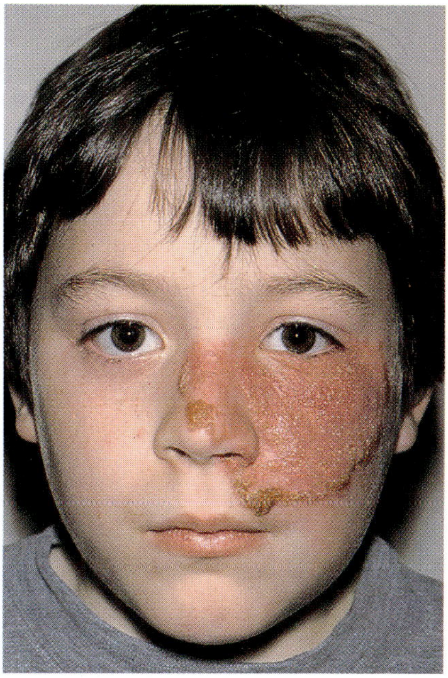

Fig. 7.5 Tinea incognito. In this extreme example of tinea treated with a potent steroid, pustules are present throughout the lesion and the edge is crusted and pustular.

clinical features of this are of a predominantly monomorphic eruption of red papules and pustules centred around hair follicles, occurring particularly on the upper trunk and upper arms (Fig. 7.6). It appears to be caused by degeneration of the follicular epithelium (Kaidbey & Kligman 1974).

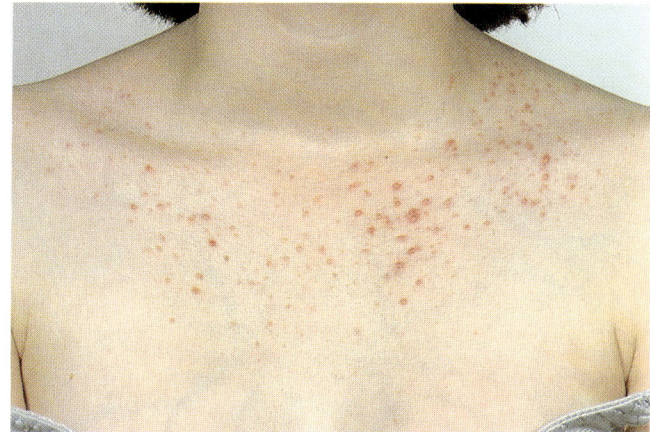

Fig. 7.6 Steroid acne. Papules and pustules precipitated by topical steroids.

'Steroid face', rosacea and peri-oral dermatitis

'Steroid face' is a striking clinical picture with marked erythema and telangiectasia which are the result partly of steroid-induced capillary dilatation and partly of loss of the vascular support tissue due to steroid-induced atrophy of dermal connective tissue. A common problem with this condition is that application of the steroid produces temporary vasoconstriction with improvement of the plethoric appearance and so the patient continues to apply the steroid for this effect, thus worsening the underlying condition. Only complete cessation of steroid applications will arrest the process and a prolonged course of tetracyclines will help to improve the appearance. In general, this condition results from the use of potent topical steroids on the face over a considerable period of time. A few people, however, seem to be particularly susceptible to the effects of steroids and will develop some degree of 'steroid face' after only a few applications of a potent or even a moderately potent preparation.

The application of potent topical steroids to the face will worsen any pre-existing rosacea (Sneddon 1969) and can precipitate a rosacea-like picture with erythema, papules, pustules and telangiectasia over the cheeks, nose and forehead (Leyden, Thew & Kligman 1974). (Fig. 7.7) This condition often overlaps with 'steroid face'.

Perioral dermatitis is a related condition (Sneddon 1972) in which erythema, papules, pustules and scaling develop in the perioral region (Fig. 7.8), usually in young females who have been ill-advisedly applying topical steroids for acne vulgaris or for mild facial eczema. A striking clinical feature is the conspicuous sparing of the vermillion border of the lips so that the mouth appears to be outlined in white. Like rosacea and 'steroid face' this condition responds to total withdrawal of topical steroids and a long course of oral tetracyclines.

Fig. 7.7 Rosacea exacerbated by topical steroid application. Striking erythema with telangiectases, purpura, papules and pustules.

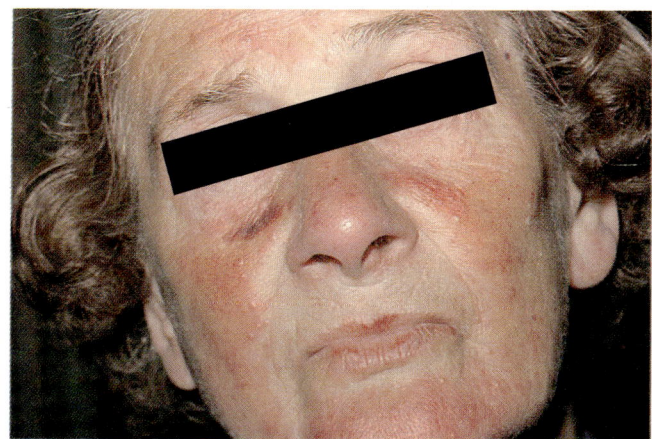

Fig. 7.8 Perioral dermatitis. Erythema, papules and pustules with sparing of the vermillion border of the lips.

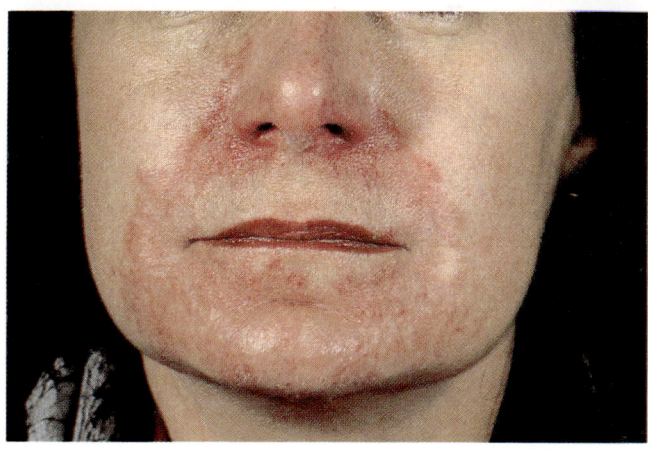

Glaucoma

Potent topical steroids should not be applied to the eyelids except under close supervision because of the risk of precipitating glaucoma.

Leucoderma

Areas of hypopigmentation and of cutaneous and subcutaneous tissue atrophy may develop at the site of intralesional (including intra-articular) steroid injections (Cahn 1979) (Fig. 7.9).

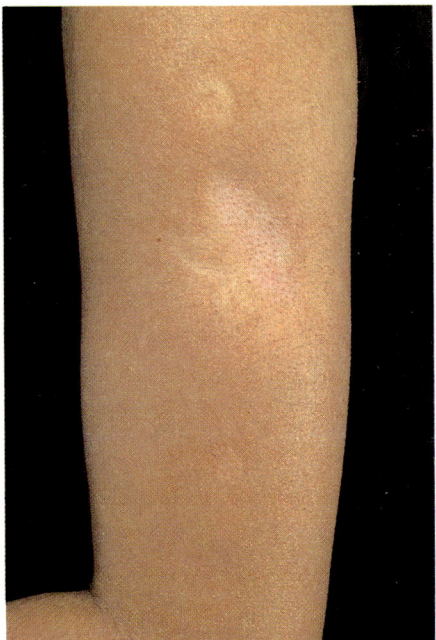 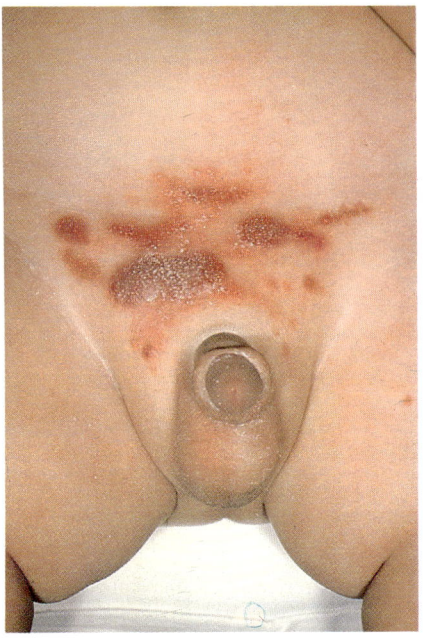

Fig. 7.9 Leucoderma and atrophy. At the site of a previous steroid injection.

Fig. 7.10 Infantile gluteal granulomata may be caused by potent steroids applied under plastic pant occlusion. Photograph courtesy of Dr D.J. Atherton, St John's Hospital for Diseases of the Skin and published with the kind permission of the Editor, *Clinical and Experimental Dermatology*.

Infantile gluteal granuloma

This condition is characterised by the development of dusky red nodules in a pre-existing napkin eruption (Fig. 7.10). The exact aetiology has not been elucidated but potent topical steroids, used to treat the initial eruption under the occlusion provided by plastic pants, are instrumental in causing the lesions (Bonifazi *et al.* 1981; Lovell & Atherton 1984). When steroid applications are stopped, the lesions resolve slowly but often leave atrophic scars.

Pustular psoriasis

It is thought that generalised pustular psoriasis, a rare but potentially fatal condition, may be provoked by abrupt cessation of treatment with potent topical steroids (Ryan & Baker 1971; Boxley, Dawber & Summerley 1975). Paradoxically, there is also evidence that pustular psoriasis may develop during treatment with potent steroids (Baker 1976). The underlying reasons for these effects have not yet been elucidated but very potent steroids should be used with caution in the treatment of psoriasis.

Allergic contact eczema

Allergic reactions to topical steroids are uncommon but well documented, the allergen usually being a preservative or other constituent of the base. However, true contact allergy to the steroid itself has been reported but is very rare (Alani & Alani 1972).

SYSTEMIC SIDE-EFFECTS

It has long been recognised that topically applied corticosteroids are absorbed through the skin with or without polythene occlusion, and that if sufficient steroid is absorbed into the circulation, hypothalamic-pituitary-adrenal (HPA) axis suppression will occur (Scoggins & Kliman 1965; James, Munro & Feiwel 1967). Iatrogenic Cushing's syndrome is still seen in patients who have applied liberal quantities of potent steroids for prolonged periods (Fig. 7.11). Systemic absorption is further enhanced by applying steroids to red, diseased skin, and by the atrophy and vasodilatation which results locally from long-term steroid use.

Nevertheless, in most cases, the suppression of hypothalamic-pituitary-adrenal function is a rever-

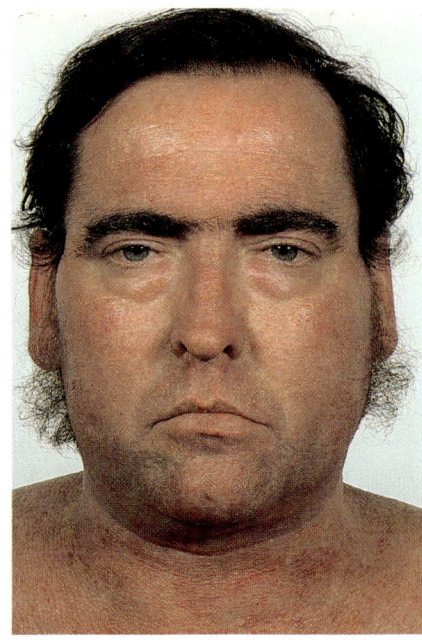

Fig. 7.11 Excessive use of a very potent steroid over many years produced Cushing's syndrome in this man.

sible biochemical finding rather than a clinical problem (James, Munro & Feiwel 1967) and many of the earlier studies reporting this effect were carried out on patients who were applying 30 g or more of potent steroid per day, often under occlusive dressings. Subsequent studies on out-patients using potent topical steroids revealed little effect on plasma corticosteroid levels (Wilson, Williams & Marsh 1973) or on adrenal axis response as determined by insulin stress tests (Munro & Clift 1973). The conclusion to be drawn is that, in sensible out-patient practice, HPA axis suppression is a theorettical rather than a practical risk when using moderately potent or potent steroids in adults. The situation is different for the very potent steroids and for children. It is not possible to lay down a limit for the amount of potent steroid which may be safely applied per week, since this depends to a large degree on the size of the patient and the state of the skin being treated. Most of the outpatients in the studies referred to above were applying less than 60 g/week with no significant effects on pituitary adrenal function. However, a sensible clinical rule is that, if a patient is regularly using 30 g or more of a potent topical steroid per week, the treatment regime should be reviewed. For example, if the patient has psoriasis it may be time to use alternative treatments such as dithranol or ultraviolet light. If the diagnosis is eczema, perhaps the treatment of infection, dry skin or pruritus needs to be increased.

The risk of HPA axis suppression is much greater with the very potent group of topical steroids such as clobetasol propionate. The application of 50 g per week of this preparation to normal skin is sufficient to produce significant HPA axis suppression (Fig. 7.12) (Carruthers, August & Staughton 1975) and less steroid is required to produce this effect when applied to diseased, erythematous skin. Absorption through the thick stratum corneum of the palms and soles is minimal, even with the use of occlusion so less caution is needed when treating these areas with very potent steroids. In general, however, the amounts of very potent steroids applied must be

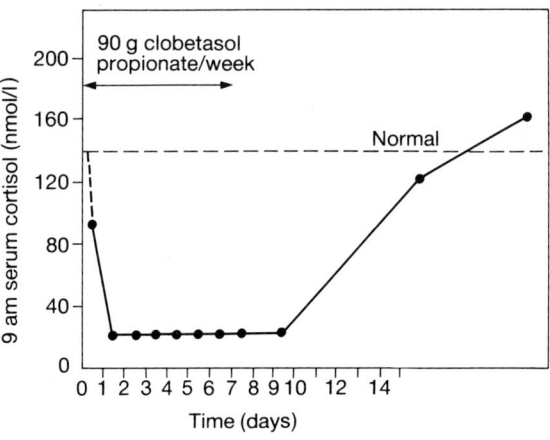

Fig. 7.12 HPA axis suppression. Response of one normal person to the application of 90 g clobetasol propionate cream weekly, to the whole body. (Carruthers *et al.* 1975)
With the kind permission of the authors and British Medical Association.

monitored carefully and patients should not be using more than 15 g per week.

Children are more susceptible than adults to the systemic side-effects of the potent topical steroids. This is partly because of the greater surface area to volume ratio in children, and partly because of increased sensitivity to small degrees of suppression of the HPA axis. Growth retardation is a particularly important consequence of steroid absorption in children (Feiwel 1969) and potent steroids should only be prescribed for children in exceptional circumstances and, preferably, only under specialist supervision. It must be emphasised, however, that hydrocortisone preparations, unless used excessively, are free from local and systemic side-effects even in children.

Special mention should be made of 0.05% clobetasone butyrate (Eumovate) which is classified as a moderately potent corticosteroid. Studies in animals and in man have shown that this compound shows a specific separation of topical from systemic activity (Munro & Wilson 1975; Marshall & du Vivier 1978). It has useful topical anti-inflammatory activity, being effective in the treatment of eczema and, to a lesser extent, psoriasis. However, it causes less thinning of the epidermis than steroids other than hydrocortisone and has a minimal effect on HPA function even under conditions predisposing to maximal percutaneous absorption.

REFERENCES

Alani M.D. & Alani S.D. (1972). Allergic contact dermatitis to corticosteroids. *Ann Allergy* **30**: 181.
Baker H. (1976). Corticosteroids and pustular psoriasis. *Br J Dermatol* **94**(12): 83.
Bonifazi E., Garofalo L., Lospallut M., Scardigno A., Corviello C. & Meneghini C.L. (1981). Granuloma gluteale infantum with atrophic scars: Clinical and histological observations in 11 cases. *Clin Exp Dermatol* **6**: 23.
Boxley J.D., Dawber R.P.R. & Summerley R. (1975). Generalised pustular psoriasis on withdrawal of clobetasol propionate ointment. *Br Med J* **2**: 255.

Cahn B.I. (1979). Leukoderma acquisitum secondary to intralesional steroid injection. *Cutis* **9**: 509.

Carruthers J.A., August P.J. & Staughton R.C.D. (1975). Observations on the systemic effect of topical clobetasol propionate (Dermovate). *Br Med J* **4**: 203.

Daltrey D.C. & Cunliffe W.J. (1983). Effect of betamethasone 17-valerate on the normal human facial skin flora. *Acta Derm Venereol* **63**: 160.

Epstein N.N., Epstein W.L. & Epstein J.H. (1963). Atrophic striae in patients with inguinal intertrigo. *Arch Dermatol* **87**: 450.

Feiwel M. (1969). Percutaneous absorption of topical steroids in children. *Br J Dermatol* **81** (4): 113.

Ive F.A. & Marks R. (1968). Tinea incognito. *Br Med J* **3**: 149.

James V.H.T., Munro D.D. & Feiwel M. (1967). Pituitary-adrenal function after occlusive topical therapy with betamethasone 17-valerate. *Lancet* **ii**: 1059.

Kaidbey K.H. & Kligman A.M. (1974). The pathogenesis of topical steroid acne. *J Invest Dermatol* **62**: 31.

Kirby J.D. & Munro D.D. (1976). Steroid-induced atrophy in an animal and human model. *Br J Dermatol* **94** (12): 111.

Leyden J.J., Thew M. & Kligman A.M. (1974). Steroid rosacea. *Arch Dermatol* **110**: 619.

Lovell C.R. & Atherton D.J. (1984). Infantile gluteal granulomata — case report. *Clin Exp Dermatol* **9**: 522.

Marshall R.C. & du Vivier A. (1978). The effects on epidermal DNA synthesis of the butyrate esters of clobetasone and clobetasol, and the propionate ester of clobetasol. *Br J Dermatol* **98**: 355.

Munro D.D. & Clift D.C. (1973). Pituitary-adrenal function after prolonged use of topical corticosteroids. *Br J Dermatol* **88**: 381.

Munro D.D. & Wilson L. (1975). Clobetasone butyrate, a new topical corticosteroid: clinical activity and effects on pituitary-adrenal axis function and model of epidermal atrophy. *Br Med J* **3**: 626.

Ryan T.J. & Baker H. (1971). The prognosis of generalized pustular psoriasis. *Br J Dermatol* **85**: 407.

Scoggins R.B. & Kliman B. (1965). Percutaneous absorption of corticosteroids — systemic effects. *N Engl J Med* **273**: 831.

Sneddon I.B. (1969). Adverse effects of topical fluorinated corticosteroids in rosacea. *Br Med J* **1**: 671.

Sneddon I.B. (1972). Perioral dermatitis. *Br J Dermatol* **87**: 430.

Wilson L., Williams D.I. & Marsh S.D. (1973). Plasma corticosteroid levels in out-patients treated with topical steroids. *Br J Dermatol* **88**: 373.

SIDE-EFFECTS

When do side-effects occur
- Inappropriate potency prescribed
- Incorrect diagnosis made
- Repeat prescriptions issued
- Too much applied by patient
- Incorrect use by patient for different eruption

Local side-effects
- Atrophy
- Masking of infection
- Acne and folliculitis
- Rosacea and perioral dermatitis
- Glaucoma
- Leucoderma
- Infantile gluteal granulomata
- Modification of psoriasis

Systemic side-effects
- HPA axis suppression
- Cushing's syndrome
- Growth retardation in children

Chapter 8
Practical Aspects of Prescribing

Some of the available topical steroid preparations consist of the steroid alone, others contain the steroid together with another active agent. In addition, ready-diluted topical steroids are available. Most of these preparations are available in more than one formulation, such as ointment, cream, or lotion, hence the writing of a single prescription involves many choices and decisions.

TOPICAL STEROID PREPARATION

Formulation

An ointment is the best formulation for most clinical situations. Ointments do not sting when applied and do not contain potential allergens such as preservatives or lanolin. Their greasiness aids penetration of the active agent and also helps to correct the dryness of the skin which often accompanies steroid-responsive disorders. However, weeping lesions are sometimes better treated with a cream or lotion until the eruption has dried. Some patients find the greasiness of ointments unacceptable and may request creams. Lotions are usually prescribed for scalp disorders to avoid excessive greasiness of the hair.

Combined preparations

Many available preparations contain another active agent with the steroid.

Emollients

Hydrocortisone with an emollient such as urea (e.g. in Alphaderm, Calmurid HC) is useful in the treatment of very dry atopic eczema.

Anti-infective agents

Antibiotic agents in combination with steroids are often useful in the treatment of infected eczema, particularly atopic eczema in children and discoid eczema in adults. The moist intertriginous areas (including the napkin area) provide favourable conditions for the growth of infection especially in the presence of a topical steroid. Hence eruptions in these areas are often best treated by a steroid combined with either an anticandidal agent or a broad spectrum anti-infective agent such as vioform (clioquinol). Particular caution must be observed when using antibiotic or anticandidal-steroid combinations in older patients because of the risk of allergic sensitisation to the anti-infective component. They should never be prescribed for varicose eczema, since sensitisation occurs particularly readily in this situation. Preparations containing hydrocortisone combined with an anti-fungal agent may occasionally be useful in the treatment of very inflammatory tinea infections. They should not, however, be used as a panacea; the diagnosis of a tinea infection should be established and treated appropriately.

Local anaesthetics

Although commercially available, the usefulness of local anaesthetic-steroid combinations is limited. They are rarely used by dermatologists and there is a considerable risk of sensitisation to the anaesthetic component, producing contact dermatitis.

Tar and dithranol

Topical steroids can also be mixed with other therapeutic agents by the dispensing pharmacist. Thus, for example, dilutions of potent topical steroids mixed with tar or with various concentrations of dithranol are valuable in the treatment of psoriasis since such therapy combines the different advantages of the topical steroid and the alternative treatments. Animal research has shown that such combinations may actually be more effective than the active compounds used alone (Clement *et al.* 1983) and patients find a mixture of steroid and dithranol a more acceptable treatment than dithranol alone.

PRESCRIBING TOPICAL STEROIDS

Quantities

When prescribing a topical steroid it is important to make some estimate of how much the patient will need and to be aware of how much the patient is actually using.

Treatment failure may be because too little has been prescribed by the doctor or used by the patient. Side-effects occur when too much is applied over too long a period.

Between 15 and 25 g of cream or ointment is required to cover the entire body of an average adult on one application. Hence it is futile to prescribed a 30 g tube for a patient with widespread eczema and expect it to last for a month. On the other hand, side-effects can be predicted if a patient is obtaining 100 g per week of a potent preparation on a repeat prescription basis. Regular monitoring of the patient's requirements is imperative. The rule of nines can be used to estimate the amounts required for small areas of the body.

Munro (1984) has suggested the following guidelines for prescribing topical steroids (*see* Table 8.1): in one week an adult may safely use 50 g of a mildly or moderately potent preparation; 30 g of a potent steroid; or 15 g of a very potent preparation. These quantities may be doubled for periods of up to two months but should be halved if treatment continues for longer than six months.

Dilutions

The choice of potency was discussed in Chapters 4–6 but what of the practice of diluting topical steroids to provide a fine adjustment to potency? There has been much discussion among members of the pharmaceutical industry and dermatologists as to the value of diluting proprietary preparations. Careful dilution with the correct diluent is an accurate technique (Clement *et al.* 1983) and does reduce unwanted effects. However, dilution with an inappropriate vehicle may inactivate the steroid and also carries, the risk of introducing microbial contamination. With the wide range of products of different potencies available, including ready-diluted preparations, the diluting of proprietary corticosteroid applications is now regarded as an unnecessary and outmoded practice.

Frequency of application

Little is known about the optimal treatment regimes for topical steroids. There is theoretical evidence that repeated application produces tolerance in the skin with diminished effectiveness, a phenomenon known as tachyphylaxis (du Viver & Stoughton 1975; Barry & Woodford 1977; du Vivier, Phillips & Hehir 1982; Clement, Phillips & du Vivier 1985). The clinical relevance of this is obscure and adequate therapeutic results are usually obtained by applying the preparation daily or, in severe eruptions, twice

Table 8.1 Safe prescribing of topical steroids: maximum weekly adult dosages (g)

Treatment period (months)	Potency		
	Mild & Moderate	Potent	Very Potent
<2	100	60	30
2–6	50	30	15
6–12	25	15	7.5

daily. There is no apparent extra benefit from more frequent applications. Once the disorder being treated is under control, treatment may be stopped or either the frequency or the potency of the treatment reduced to obtain adequate suppression of the disease process. When potent steroids are being used to treat a chronic condition such as psoriasis, intermittent short courses are preferable so the side-effects are minimised. Bland preparations should be applied between treatments for their emollient effect.

Patients frequently report that their skin disease becomes resistant to one steroid preparation and that changing to another steroid even within the same potency group produces a renewed beneficial effect. It is possible that this is a practical manifestation of the phenomenon of tachyphylaxis.

Method of application

Patients should always be instructed to apply topical steroids sparingly: a thick covering of ointment does not guarantee more effective or faster recovery and only increases the likelihood of side-effects. If a potent steroid is being used or if treatment is likely to be long term, the patient should be advised to keep a record of the amounts of steroid applied. Regular review is preferable to repeat prescriptions when possible and the very potent steroids should never be supplied on a repeat prescription basis.

Occlusive techniques are valuable because they keep the application on the skin and prevent it from being rubbed off onto clothes or bedclothes. They also aid penetration of the steroid and polythene occlusion is particularly useful for treating resistant eruptions on the palms and soles. Patients may use clingwrap or plastic bags tied round the wrists and ankles or obtain plastic disposable gloves from large chemists. The use of polythene occlusion at other sites, however, carries an increased risk of adverse effects (Chapter 7).

Occlusion by bandaging is useful in treating pruritic skin disorders since it reduces access to the skin and hence the traumatic effects of scratching which perpetuate the disease. Atopic eczema, lichen simplex and nodular prurigo are particular examples of diseases which benefit from bandaging. The bandages used may be plain (e.g. crepe) or medicated, containing another therapeutic agent such as zinc, tar or ichthammol.

An interesting and useful method of delivery of steroid to the skin is in the form of an adhesive tape; flurandrenolone (Haelan) tape. This supplies a moderately potent steroid under occlusion and is often effective in treating discoid lupus erythematosus, granulomatous conditions such as granuloma annulare and the lesions of nodular prurigo and lichen simplex.

Finally, intralesional steroids are useful in the management of many skin disorders, particularly lichen simplex, nodular prurigo, alopecia areata, hypertrophic scars and the granulomatous conditions. The injection may be made either via multiple puncture sites with an instrument such as a Dermojet or through a fine needle attached to an insulin syringe. Care must be taken to inject into the lesion and not into the subcutis since unsightly atrophy may result.

REFERENCES

Barry B. & Woodford R. (1977). Vasoconstrictor activities and bio-availabilities of seven proprietary corticosteroid creams assessed using a non-occluded multiple dosage regimen; clinical implications. *Br J Dermatol* **97**: 555.

Clement M., Hehir M., Phillips H. & du Vivier A. (1983). The effect on epidermal DNA synthesis of a combination of topical steroid with either dithranol or tar as used for psoriasis. *Br J Dermatol* **109**: 327.

Clement M., Phillips H. & du Vivier A. (1985). Is steroid tachyphylaxis preventable? *Clin Exp Dermatol* **10**: 22.

du Vivier A., Phillips H. & Hehir M. (1982). Applications of glucocorticosteroids: The effects of twice-daily vs once-every-other-day applications on mouse epidermal DNA synthesis. *Arch Dermatol* **118**: 305.

du Vivier A. & Stoughton R.B. (1975). Tachyphylaxis to the action of topically applied corticosteroids. *Arch Dermatol* **111**: 581.

Munro D.D. (1984). The graded use of topical steroids. *Perspect Ther N Eur* **18**: 5.

EFFECTIVE PRESCRIBING OF TOPICAL STEROIDS

- Precise instructions to patient: how often, how much, where to, how long for
- Appropriate potency and formulation
- Other aspects of management, e.g. emollients, antibiotics, antihistamines
- Combined preparations may be useful
- Monitor quantities used by patient
- No repeat prescriptions for more potent steroids

Index

Acne, steroid produced   23, 26, **52−3**
Acne vulgaris   23, 24, 27, 52, 54
Action of steroids   **9−14**
Adcortyl   17
Age, effects of   27, **29−31**, 32, 33
Allergic contact eczema, *see* Eczema
Alopecia areata   18, **47**, 68
Alphaderm   17, 18, 64
Aluminium acetate soaks   37, 38
Angio-oedema   13
Antibiotics   28, 33, 34, 35, 36, 37, 38, 40, 41, 64
Antihistamines   34, 38, 41, 46
Anti-inflammatory effects   1, **9−10, 12**, 14, 16, 40, 42, 60
Anti-mitotic effects   **11−12, 13**, 16, 42
Application frequency   **66−7**
Application methods   **67−8**
Asteatotic eczema, *see* Eczema
Atopic eczema, *see* Eczema
Atrophy   25, 28, 29, 30, 36, 47, **49−51**, 55, 56, 57, 68

Bandaging   19, 34, 46, 68
Beclomethasone dipropionate (Propaderm)   17
Betamethasone 17-valerate (Betnovate)   2−3, **5, 7**, 8, 16, 17, 19, 51
Betnovate, *see* Betamethasone 17-valerate
Blanching effect   2, 16
Blood supply, and absorption   21

Calmurid HC   17, 18, 64
Candida infection   25, 40, 41, 51, 64
Children
  eczema in, *see* Eczema
  psoriasis in, *see* Psoriasis
  risks to   19, **29−30**, 31, 58, 60
Clioquinol   64
Clobetasol propionate (Dermovate)   3, 5, 7, 8, 17, 44, 59, 60
Clobetasone butyrate (Eumovate)   1, 7, 60
Combined steroid-anti-infective preparation   34, 36, 37, 40, 41, 64

Contact dermatitis, *see* Eczema
Corticotropin   1, 5
Cortisone   1, 5, 6
Creams   19, 28, 36, 40, 63, 65
Cushing's syndrome   3, 57, 58

Dermatitis, *see* Eczema
Dermovate, *see* Clobetasol propionate
Diflucortolone valerate (Nerisone)   17
Dilution of steroids   66
Dinitrochlorobenzene   11
Discoid eczema, *see* Eczema
Discoid lupus erythematosus   12, 18, 24, **46**, 68
Dithranol   42, 44, 59, 65
DNA synthesis suppression   12, 17

Eczema (dermatitis)   1, 3, 5, 12, 17, 18, **32−41**, 50, 51, 59, 60
  allergic contact/contact dermatitis   24, 28, **41, 57**, 63, 64
  asteatotic/eczema craquelé   **39**, 40
  atopic   23, 27, 29, **32−5**, 48, 64, 68
  in children   18, **29−30**, 32, 33, 36, 40, 41, 64
  discoid   18, 30, **37**, 48, 64
  facial   18, 22, 23, 24, **35**, 54
  of flexures   18, **25**, 35, 36
  genital   25, **40**
  of hands and feet   18, **28**, 33, 37, 38, 48
  impetiginised/infected   **32−6**, 64
  of limbs   18, **27−8**, 30, 32, 33, 34, 36, 37
  napkin dermatitis   29, 30, **40**
  perioral   54, 55
  pompholyx   38
  primary irritant   28, **38−40**, 41
  of scalp   **25−6**
  seborrhoeic   **34−6**
    of infancy   29, **36**
  of trunk   18, 30, 33, 35
  varicose   28, **36**, 37, 64
Efcortelan   17
Elderly, risks to   30, 31, 64
Emollients   34, 36, 38, 39, 40, 64, 67
Erythema   29, 35, 54, 55
Erythrasma   25

Index

Esterification 7, 8, 18
Eumovate, see Clobetasone butyrate

Face 18, 19, 21, **22−4**, 31, 33, 34, 35, 42, 46, 54, 55
Feet 18, 21, 27, **28**, 31, 33, 37, 44, 59, 68
Flexural areas 18, 19, 21, **25**, 30, 31, 35, 36, 42, 43, 50
Fluocinolone acetonide (Synalar and Synandone) 1, 5, 8, 16, 17
Fluocinonide (Metosyn) 17
Flurandrenolone (Haelan) 17
Flurandrenolone tape (Haelan tape) 68
Fluorination 7, 8, 54
Folliculitis 28, 51, 52
Formulation 8, 19, **63**
Fungal infections 51−2, 64
 see also Candida; Tinea

Genitalia 21, **25**, 40, 41
Glaucoma **55**
Granuloma annulare **47**, 68
Growth retardation 29, 60

Haelan, see Flurandrenolone
Haelan tape, see Flurandrenolone tape
Hair follicle density 21
Halcinonide (Halciderm) 17
Hands 18, 21, 27, **28**, 31, 33, 37, 38, 39, 43, 44, 48, 59, 68
Hydrocortisone 1, 5, 6, 8, **18−19**, 23−4, 26, 29, 32, 33, 35, 36, 40, 60
Hydrocortisone acetate 16, 17
Hydrocortisone butyrate (Locoid) 7, 8, 17, 18
Hydrocortistab 17
Hydroxylation 7, 8
Hypothalamic-pituitary-adrenal axis suppression 19, 29, **57−60**

Ichthammol 68
Immunosuppressive effects **10−11**, 12
Impetiginised eczema see Eczema
Infantile gluteal granuloma 30, **56**
Infantile seborrhoeic eczema see Eczema
Infected eczema see Eczema
Infection, masking of **50−2**
Infection, secondary 28, 29, 32−3, 34, 35, 36, 37, 40, 51, 64
Inflammatory response 10
Inguinal intertrigo 50
Insect bites 12, 48
Intralesional steroids 45, 46, 47, 48, 55, 56, 68

Isopropyl myristate 8

Keloid scars 48
Keratolytic preparations 26, 43, 44
Leucoderma 55, 56
Lichen planus 12, 13, 18, 19, **44**
Lichen simplex 18, **45**, **46**, 68
Limbs 18, **27−8**, 30, 31, 33, 34, 36, 37, 53
Lipomodulin 10, 11
Local anaesthetics 64
Local side-effects **49−57**
Locoid, see Hydrocortisone butyrate
Lotions 19, 63

Macrocortin 10, 11
Masking of infection 50−2
Methylation 7, 8
Metosyn, see Fluocinonide

Napkin dermatitis see Eczema
Necrobiosis lipoidica 47
Nerisone Forte 17
Nodular prurigo **45, 46**, 68

Occlusion 3, 19, 21, 25, 28, 34, 40, 44, 51, 56, 57, 58, 59, 68
Ointments 19, 63, 65, 67

Patch testing 24, 40, 48
Percutaneous absorption 19, 21, 22, 23, 28, 31, 57, 59−60, 68
Perioral dermatitis, see Eczema
Phospholipase A_2 10, 11
Pityriasis rosea 26
Pityriasis versicolor 26, 27, 51−2
Polythene occlusion 3, 28, 44, 51, 57, 68
Pompholyx, see Eczema
Potassium permanganate 38
Potency groups 16, 17
 and prescription 66
Prednisolone 6, 7
Prescribing steroids 63, **65−8**, 69
 inappropriate 18, 26, 34, 49, 50, 51
Primary irritant eczema, see Eczema
Propaderm, see Beclomethasone dipropionate
Propylene glycol 19
Prurigo nodularis see Nodular prurigo
Pruritus 13, 33, 59, 68
Psoriasis 3, 5, 10, 14, 18, **42−4**, **48**, 60, 65, 67

in children 30, 44
facial 18, 23, 42
of flexures 18, 25, 30, 42, 43
genital 25
of hands and feet 28, 43
pustular **57**
of scalp 26, 42, 43
Purpura 20, 28, 29, 30, 36, 51, 55
Pustular psoriasis, *see* Psoriasis

Rosacea 15, 25, 54, 55

Salicylic acid 19
Sarcoidosis 47
Scabies 27, 51
Scalp **25–6**, 35, 36, 42, 43, 47, 63, 65
Scars 48, 56, 68
Scrotum 21, 25
Seborrhoeic eczema, *see* Eczema
Secondary infection, *see* Infection, secondary
Side-effects of topical steroids 3, 14, 18, 19, 25, 26, 27, 28, 30, 35, 42, **49–60**, 65, 68
Skin, thickness of 21, 22, 23, 25
thickened areas 18, 28, 44, 45, 59
thinning of 14, 28, **50**, 51, 60
Solar keratoses 26
Staphylococcal infection 33, 50
Steroid acne 23, 26, **52–3**
'Steroid face' 15, **54**
Steroid purpura 20, 28, 29, 30, 50, 55
Steroid vehicle 8

Striae 25, 28, 36, 49, 50, 51
Structural modification **6–8**
Sunburn 12, 48
Synalar 17
Synandone 17
Systemic side-effects **57–60**

Tachyphylaxis 66–7
Tape, adhesive 68
Tar 26, 35, 42, 44, **65**, 68
Telangiectasia 30, 50, 54, 55
Tetracyclines 54
Tinea 25, 28, 52, 53, 64
Tinea incognito 52, 53
Triamcinolone acetonide 1, 5, 7, 8, 17, 44
Trunk 18, **26–7**, 30, 33, 35, 53

Ulceration 27, 30, 36, 51
Ultraviolet light treatment 44, 59
Urea 17, 18, 19, 64
Urticaria 13

Varicose eczema, *see* Eczema
Vasoconstriction 2, **12, 14**, 16, 54, 57
Vasoconstictor assay 1, 2, 16
Vasodilation 12, 57
Vioform 64
Viral infections 34

Zinc 68